# POCKET GUIDE TO MUSCULOSKELETAL ASSESSMENT

## RICHARD E. BAXTER, MPT

Chief of Physical Therapy
Munson Army Health Center
Fort Leavenworth, Kansas

## W.B. SAUNDERS COMPANY

An *Imprint of Elsevier Science*
Philadelphia  London  New York  St. Louis  Sydney  Toronto

**W.B. SAUNDERS COMPANY**

*An Imprint of Elsevier Science*

The Curtis Center
Independence Square West
Philadelphia, Pennsylvania 19106

### Library of Congress Cataloging-in-Publication Data

Baxter, Richard, MPT.

Pocket guide to musculoskeletal assessment / Richard Baxter.

p.    cm.

ISBN 0–7216–3337–4

1. Musculoskeletal system—Diseases—Diagnosis—Handbooks,
    manuals, etc.    I. Title.
    [DNLM: 1. Musculoskeletal Diseases—diagnosis—handbooks.
    2. Physical Examination—methods—handbooks.
    WE 39 B355m 1998]

RC925.7.B39 1998      616.7′075—dc21

DNLM/DLC                                                       97-18626

The author is a physical therapist in the United States Army and is currently the Chief of Physical Therapy at Munson Army Health Center, Fort Leavenworth, Kansas. The views presented are those of the author and do not necessarily represent the views of the Department of Defense or its components.

To the Creator of this amazing body
that we study and attempt to comprehend,
who has blessed me beyond what
I could have ever imagined.

# PREFACE

This project began with one goal: easing the stress and burden of clinical affiliations as a physical therapy student. I envisioned accomplishing this by providing myself a framework for performing thorough neuromusculoskeletal evaluations, including accessible quick reference tables for special tests and possible treatment options. I wanted it to be compact, so that I could carry it in a lab coat pocket. Since I rarely had time during patient care to go back and study a textbook, this quick reference book came in very handy.

Never in my wildest dream did I imagine that this personal project would be published. As classmates saw its value and wanted copies for themselves, instructors and other physical therapists also noted that it was a very useful tool in the clinical setting. The book grew and changed over time to take on its present form. Had I known beforehand the tremendous amount of research, organization, revision, energy, and hours that would be required, I would surely have been overwhelmed.

This is not a comprehensive text. It is meant to provide a framework, quick reference information, reminders of how to conduct special tests, and options that may be used in developing treatment plans. I get great satisfaction in organizing/simplifying large amounts of information to make others' jobs easier. My genuine desire is that this book will be a very useful tool that makes your job easier, whether as a student or as a practicing health care provider performing neuromusculoskeletal evaluations.

I want to thank everyone who contributed to this book. I certainly did not do this on my own. In addition to everyone that I have listed by name in my acknowledgments, I would like to thank the editors and staff of the W.B. Saunders Company for their support, encouragement, and tremendous assistance.

RICHARD BAXTER

# ACKNOWLEDGMENTS

So many individuals have contributed to this project that it is difficult to know where to begin. I'd like to thank Randy Sullivan, who had some evaluation outlines on index cards, for the permission to use something similar and expand the idea. I'd also like to thank Sandy Quillen for seeing the value in this text and encouraging me to publish it.

Additionally, I extend my sincere appreciation to Terry Randall, John Halle, Frank Underwood, Sandy Quillen, and Glenn Williams for the amount of time and effort that they expended reviewing the manuscript and making recommendations.

Finally, I would like to thank my classmates from physical therapy school for their contributions and encouragement in this endeavor. They include Mary Adams, Cara (Papahronis) Baldwin, Anthony Bare, Gino Chincarini, Mark Deysher, Roger Dougherty, Dave Johnson, Jonelle Jozwiak, Maire McAnaw, Lyle McClune, Tammy McKenzie, Glen Myatt, Allyson Pritchard, Tami Roehr, Susan Romito, Chu Soh, Jeff Struebing, Kathy Vrydaghs, Bryan Whitesides, Julie Whitman, and Glenn Williams.

RICHARD BAXTER

# CONTENTS

# 1

# INTRODUCTION

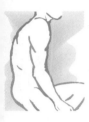

**KISS:** "Keep It Super Simple." KISS is the essence of this quick reference guide to neuromusculoskeletal evaluations and treatment options for some common conditions encountered in the clinic. This is neither a comprehensive text nor an attempt to capture all aspects of physical therapy and reduce them to fit a pocket handbook. This guide is meant to provide only a framework for a thorough neuromusculoskeletal evaluation and treatment. I hope you will use this guide, as I do, to keep patient examinations organized, efficient, and thorough. When examining a patient, you may find it helpful to open the guide to the body region in question and lay the book on the nearest available flat surface.

Located at the beginning of each section is **S/Pt Hx** for subjective/patient history/profile and **O** for objective, which are portions of the **SOAGP** note format. The **A** (assessment), **G** (goals), and **P** (plan) are left up to you, the evaluator, but the treatment options portion of each section is meant to assist in these areas. While examining a patient, you may find it necessary to glance at the outline to maintain an efficient, organized thought flow. If the correct procedure for performing a special test slips your mind during the examination, turn to the material after the outline to refresh your memory. Although there are many more special tests and modifications of the tests I have included, this handbook provides a basic group of commonly used special tests; you should feel free to write in other tests that you use in your practice.

The treatment options are, in fact, *options;* they offer only a starting point. There are many more treatment regimens, protocols, and techniques than could be presented in this text. In some cases, I included tools for diagnosis or treatment that may be beyond the scope of practice for the providers using this text. For example, physical therapists within my scope of practice are credentialed to order radiographs, although this is outside the scope of practice for many, as may be the case for treatment options that include the prescription of NSAIDs. In some instances, I have included options that only a physician or surgeon may consider, such as injection or surgery. These ideas about the continuum of care may be helpful in patient education or useful as a reminder of the various options available to the patient who is referred for further intervention.

Basic outlines for respiratory, cardiac, amputee, neurologic, and acute inpatient evaluations are given to help in acute care settings. To save space, many standard terms are abbreviated throughout the book. These are explained in Appendix K.

My sincere hope is that this guide is a useful tool for you in the clinic and that it motivates you to continued study, learning, and growth. Many physical therapy and physician assistant students, as well as practicing physical therapists and physician assistants, have found it to be helpful, and I believe you will too!

## Subjective Examination

Although not exhaustive, the following is the framework for the subjective examination used in the evaluation outlines throughout the text. Only those items that are most pertinent to each region have been included in an abbreviated format in the specific body region subjective examination outlines.

▶ Age
▶ Sex
▶ Chief complaint
▶ Onset of Sx (insidious, from trauma or overuse)
▶ Body chart (body diagram with location of Sx, depth/quality/type of pain, whether pain is constant/intermittent, interaction between pain sites, presence of paresthesia)
▶ Duration of Sx (if insidious)
▶ MOI (if due to trauma)
▶ Nature of pain (constant/intermittent, deep/superficial, boring/sharp/stabbing/hot/ache, AM/PM difference in the Sx, sclerotomal or dermatomal pattern) *(see Appendices A and B)*
▶ AGG (positions or activities, how long it takes to aggravate Sx and how long to recover)
▶ Easing factors (what relieves Sx)
▶ Radiographs/CT scans/MRI/lab results
▶ Meds
▶ Occupation/recreation/hobbies
▶ Diet/tobacco/alcohol
▶ Exercise
▶ $PMH_x$ (e.g., H/O cancer, cardiovascular disease, HTN, adult/child illnesses)
▶ $PSH_x$
▶ Family history
▶ Review of systems and SQ
  ▮ General health/last physical examination
  ▮ Unexplained weight loss
  ▮ Night pain
  ▮ Bilateral extremity numbness/tingling
  ▮ Systems*

*Region-specific questions are located in applicable evaluation outlines.

1 INTRODUCTION

Skin                     Musculoskeletal

Endocrine                Pulmonary

Cardiovascular           Lymphatic

Gastrointestinal         Neurologic

Urinary/reproductive

▶ Patient's goals

# Objective Examination

Although not exhaustive, the following is the framework for the objective examination used in the evaluation outlines throughout the text. Only those positions and items that are most pertinent to each region have been included in an abbreviated format in each region-specific evaluation outline.

## Position Sequence

I. Standing

II. Sitting

III. Supine

IV. Sidelying

V. Prone

## Items to Assess in Each Position as Applicable

I. R/O other pathology by "clearing" joint above and below or other areas that refer similar Sx*

II. Observation

  A. Gait (e.g., cadence, stride length, weight bearing, antalgic, base of support, sequence)

*For the musculoskeletal screening examination of adjacent joints, apply only the most sensitive tests for the most common musculoskeletal abnormalities. Check AROM, PROM, GMMT. The purpose is to assist in detecting all areas of involvement or additional findings that may alter the diagnosis.

    B. Posture
    C. Abnormalities, deformities, muscular atrophy
    D. Function

III. AROM *(see Appendix D)*

IV. GMMT or myotomal screen

V. Special tests (per specific region)

VI. Sensation (e.g., light touch, vibration, hot/cold, sharp/dull, two-point discrimination)

VII. Palpation (e.g., defects, pain, spasm, edema/effusion, tissue density)

VIII. Joint play (per Magee[1] and Maitland[2])

## References

1. Magee DJ: *Orthopedic Physical Assessment,* 3rd ed. Philadelphia, WB Saunders, 1997.
2. Maitland GD: *Peripheral Manipulation,* 3rd ed. Boston, Butterworth-Heinemann, 1991.

# 2

# CERVICAL SPINE

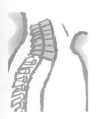

## Subjective Examination

▶ **Pt Hx (region specific):** nature of pain (dermatomal or sclerotomal)? *(see Appendices A and B)*

▶ Does coughing, sneezing, straining, or anything that increases intradiscal and intrathecal pressure aggravate the Sx?

▶ SQ: bilateral UE numbness and tingling, recent onset of headache, dizziness/visual disturbance/nausea, difficulty swallowing

▶ Type of work and posture/positions assumed at work, sleeping positions, type and number of pillows used

▶ Trauma? If so, was there loss of consciousness?

▶ Review of systems (endocrine, neurologic, cardiovascular, pulmonary, gastrointestinal)

# Objective Examination

I. Standing
  A. Observation
    1. Posture: structure and alignment in three planes
II. Sitting
  A. R/O shoulder or thoracic spine pathology
  B. Observation
    1. Posture (C5 or C6 radiculitis/radiculopathy tends to feel better with the arm resting overhead; C7 radiculitis/radiculopathy tends to feel better with the arm cradled against the abdomen)
      a. Forward head
      b. Rounded shoulders
      c. Protracted scapulae and other signs
  C. AROM (note quality, rhythm, pain, assessed by estimation, inclinometer, or other methods; apply overpressure, if necessary, to these motions)
    1. Cervical flex
    2. Cervical ext
    3. Cervical sidebending
    4. Cervical rot
    5. Combined motions (e.g., chin tuck, sidebending with rot)
  D. Myotomal screen and GMMT
    1. Neck flex (C1–C2)
    2. Shoulder elevation/shrug (C3–C4)
    3. Shoulder abd (C5)
    4. Elbow flex/wrist ext (C6)
    5. Elbow ext/wrist flex (C7)
    6. Thumb IP joint ext/finger flex (C8)
    7. Finger add (T1)
  E. MSRs

1. Biceps (C5)
2. Brachioradialis (C6)
3. Triceps (C7)
F. Pathologic reflexes: Hoffmann's sign
G. Special tests (as applicable)
   1. Foraminal encroachment: compression (Spurling's) test, distraction test
   2. Thoracic outlet syndrome: Adson's maneuver, costoclavicular syndrome test, hyperabduction test, Halstead's maneuver, Allen's test
   3. VA test
H. Sensation: dermatomes *(see Appendix A)*
III. Supine
A. Special tests: upper limb tension testing
B. Joint play: lat and anterior glides, cervical distraction
IV. Prone
A. Palpation: bony landmarks and soft tissue
B. Joint play
   1. PACVP
   2. PAUVP
   3. Transverse pressure
   4. Lat glides

2 | CERVICAL SPINE

# SPECIAL TESTS FOR THE CERVICAL SPINE

| Test | Detects | Test Procedure | Positive Sign |
|---|---|---|---|
| Compression (Spurling's) test[1] | Foraminal encroachment | Pt sitting and laterally flexes cervical spine to one side. Examiner presses straight down on Pt's head. This procedure is repeated on opposite side. | Pt experiences radicular pain that radiates into arm toward which head/cervical spine is flexed |
| Distraction test[1] | Foraminal encroachment | Pt sitting. Examiner places one hand under Pt's chin and other hand around occiput. Examiner slowly lifts Pt's head. | Pain in neck and into UE is relieved or decreased when cervical spine is distracted |
| Quadrant position[2] | Foraminal encroachment | Pt sitting. Pt performs combined ext, lat flex, and rot. This reduces size of intervertebral foramen. | Pain radiates into arm toward which head/cervical spine is extended, laterally flexed, and rotated |
| | | | Reproduction of Pt's Sx |
| | | | Have Pt keep eyes open to observe nystagmus if it occurs (indicative of VA compression, causing lack of blood supply to brain stem and cerebellum) |

**Vertebral artery test/neck ext-rot test[3]**

| | | | |
|---|---|---|---|
| Test 1 | VA compression or occlusion | Pt sitting and places cervical spine in combined ext and rot such that Pt is looking back over shoulder. Pt must keep eyes open. This is performed to each side for 20 sec. | Rapid eye movements, pupils dilate, dizziness, syncope, lightheadedness Controversy exists in medical community concerning this test. Some suggest that it possesses low sensitivity.[4] *Apply at your own risk*, and use caution with this test. Examiner should first have Pt perform cervical rot to see if this produces Sx of VA insufficiency before proceeding to described test position. |
| Test 2 | Rules out inner ear as cause of dizziness | Pt standing. Examiner stabilizes Pt's head by holding Pt's head with hands. Pt then rotates trunk and holds maximum rot for 20 sec to each side. | Same as for test 1 If Sx were not induced, cause of dizziness was most likely not an inner ear problem |
| Upper limb tension test (brachial plexus tension test)[5] (median nerve bias) | Dural/meningeal irritation or nerve root impingement (similar to SLR test in LE) | Pt supine. Examiner takes Pt's UE into glenohumeral abd (110 deg approx), forearm supination, wrist and finger ext, shoulder ER (90 deg approx), elbow ext and neck lat flex away from testing side. | Radicular pain/paresthesia into tested UE |

*Continued* ▶

## SPECIAL TESTS FOR THE CERVICAL SPINE Continued

| Test | Detects | Test Procedure | Positive Sign |
|------|---------|----------------|---------------|
| Upper limb tension test (brachial plexus tension test)[5] (Radial nerve bias) | Dural/meningeal irritation or nerve root impingement (similar to SLR test in LE) | Pt supine. Examiner depresses Pt's shoulder, extends elbow, flexes Pt's thumb into palm, pronates forearm, and ulnarly deviates wrist. | Radicular pain/paresthesia into tested UE |
| Upper limb tension test (brachial plexus tension test)[5] (ulnar nerve bias) | Dural/meningeal irritation or nerve root impingement (similar to SLR test in LE) | Pt supine. Examiner depresses Pt's shoulder, pronates forearm, extends wrist, flexes elbow, and abducts arm. | Radicular pain/paresthesia into tested UE |
| Hoffmann's sign[6] (pathologic reflex for UE similar to Babinski sign for LE) | Corticospinal tract lesion of spinal cord | Examiner grasps and stabilizes Pt's hand and "flicks" distal phalanx of middle finger in direction of ext (causing a quick stretch of finger flexors) | Induced flex of thumb and other fingers |
| Thoracic outlet syndrome | See Shoulder Special Tests and Thoracic Outlet Syndrome Tests table in Chapter 3 | | |

| Special Condition | Hx/Symptoms | Signs/Objective Findings | Treatment Options |
|---|---|---|---|
| Acute cervical radiculitis or radiculopathy (may be caused by disc bulge/HNP or narrowing of intervertebral foramen) | C5-C6 and C6-C7 nerve roots commonly involved<br>Radicular Sx in UE with distal paresthesia<br>Usually distal Sx worse than proximal | If in lower cervical spine, Pt feels better with arm held close to abdomen. If in upper cervical spine, Pt feels better with forearm resting overhead.<br>Objective neurologic signs with radiculopathy (decreased MSRs, UE muscle weakness) | *Acute:* relative rest, ice/heat, may consider cervical collar for 2–3 days for Pt comfort (but not more than a few days), sustained cervical traction, Pt education (neck care)<br>Goal is to centralize Sx<br>Check neurologic system each visit<br>Advise Pt that Sx may not improve for 7–10 days<br>Address posture<br>*Subacute:* Begin AROM in a painfree range<br>*Chronic:* AROM, cervical isometrics<br>Refer Pt to orthopedic surgeon or neurosurgeon for progressive neurologic deficit |

*Continued*

## TREATMENT OPTIONS FOR THE CERVICAL SPINE *Continued*

| Special Condition | Hx/Symptoms | Signs/Objective Findings | Treatment Options |
|---|---|---|---|
| Cervical spondylosis (DDD) | C5–C6 and C6–C7 most commonly involved<br>Nerve root/spinal cord pressure common from foraminal encroachment and spinal stenosis, resulting in radicular Sx | AM stiffness that is eased with movement but worsens later in day with continued activity<br>Radiograph may confirm and show decreased disc space and osteophytes/spurring | AROM exercises several times per day<br>Cervical isometrics (painfree)<br>Cervical traction (intermittent)<br>Moist heat<br>Pt education (neck care/self-treatment |
| Cervical DJD (involves facet joints) | Upper cervical<br>Gradual onset<br>Forward head posture<br>Crepitus | Pain and stiffness with rest that improves with movement<br>AROM: rot and lat flex most limited<br>Palpable thickening of facet joint margins<br>Radiograph may confirm | AROM exercises several times per day<br>Cervical isometrics (painfree)<br>Cervical traction (intermittent)<br>Moist heat<br>Pt education (neck care/self-treatment<br>Soft tissue mobilization |

| | | First, ensure Pt is stable/no Fx |
|---|---|---|
| Muscle strain or contusion | Muscle pain/soreness<br>Hx of trauma/overuse<br>Tender soft tissue with palpation<br>AROM limited by pain | *Acute:* Relative rest, ice for first 48–72 hours, moist heat with interferential electrical stimulation or ultrasound with electrical stimulation after initial 72 hours, add AROM to tolerance<br><br>*Subacute/chronic:* AROM, SCM and upper trapezius stretching, shoulder rolls, cervical isometrics (painfree), postural education |
| Acute torticollis ("wry neck")<br><br>From acute facet locking | Hx of unexpected movement or prolonged prone lying with head rotated to one side<br>Sharp pain that is unilateral and well localized<br>Protective deformity of lat flex and rot away from pain<br>Muscle guarding<br>Neurologic system: normal | *Acute:* supine lying to unload facet, ice, gentle manual distraction in line with deformity<br>Gentle PROM away from painful side<br>Cervical collar for 2–3 days to unload facets<br><br>*Subacute/chronic:* muscle energy techniques to regain AROM, progress to cervical isometrics |

*Continued* ▶

15

## TREATMENT OPTIONS FOR THE CERVICAL SPINE *Continued*

| Special Condition | Hx/Symptoms | Signs/Objective Findings | Treatment Options |
|---|---|---|---|
| Discogenic type | Pt awakens with pain<br>Sharp pain at medial border of scapula | Protective deformity of lat flex and rot away from pain<br>Muscle guarding<br>Neurologic system: normal<br>Sx increased with flex more than ext<br>Greater painfree AROM in a non–weight-bearing Pt | *Acute:* requires caution (resolves slower), relative rest, ice, sustained manual traction in line with deformity<br>Cervical collar for 2–3 days<br>Avoid cervical flex in acute stage<br>*Subacute/chronic:* AROM exercises<br>Cervical isometrics<br>Postural education |
| VA-basilar artery insufficiency | Dizziness with turning or extending head<br>Facial numbness and tingling<br>Double or blurred vision<br>Nausea/vomiting<br>Nystagmus, blackouts, tinnitus, headache | Positive VA test (should perform before initiating cervical traction or cervical mobilization)<br>Must differentiate from<br>Inner ear dysfunction<br>Multiple sclerosis and other demyelinating diseases<br>Hypo/hypertension<br>Diabetes | Refer Pt to MD |

## References

1. Magee DJ: *Orthopedic Physical Assessment,* 3rd ed. Philadelphia, WB Saunders, 1997.

2. Bland JH: *Disorders of the Cervical Spine: Diagnosis and Medical Management,* 2nd ed. Philadelphia, WB Saunders, 1994.

3. Maitland GD: *Vertebral Manipulation,* 4th ed. Boston, Butterworths, 1973.

4. Cote P, Kreitz BG, Cassidy JD, Thiel H: The validity of the extension-rotation test as a clinical screening procedure before neck manipulation: A secondary analysis. J Manipulative Physiol Ther 19:159–164, 1996.

5. Butler DS: The upper limb tension test revisited. In Grant R (ed): *Physical Therapy of the Cervical and Thoracic Spine,* 2nd ed. New York, Churchill Livingstone, 1994.

6. Kandell ER, Schwartz JH, Jessell TM (eds): *Principles of Neural Science,* 3rd ed. New York, Elsevier Science Publishing, 1991.

## Bibliography

Hertling D, Kessler RM: *Management of Common Musculoskeletal Disorders: Physical Therapy Principles and Methods,* 2nd ed. Philadelphia, JB Lippincott, 1990.

Highland TR, Dreisinger TE, Vie LL, et al: Changes in isometric strength and range of motion of the isolated cervical spine after eight weeks of clinical rehabilitation. Spine 17(Supplement 6):S77–S82, 1992.

Jones H, Jones M, Maitland GD: Examination and treatment by passive movement. In Grant R (ed): *Physical Therapy of the Cervical and Thoracic Spine,* 2nd ed. New York, Churchill Livingstone, 1994.

Kisner C, Colby LA: *Therapeutic Exercise: Foundations and Techniques,* 2nd ed. Philadelphia, FA Davis, 1990.

Magarey ME: Examination of the cervical and thoracic spine. In Grant R (ed): *Physical Therapy of the Cervical and Thoracic Spine,* 2nd ed. New York, Churchill Livingstone, 1994.

Saunders HD, Saunders R: *Evaluation, Treatment and Prevention of Musculoskeletal Disorders: Spine,* 3rd ed, vol 1. Chaska, Minnesota, Educational Opportunities, 1993.

# 3

# SHOULDER

## Subjective Examination

▶ **Pt Hx (region specific):** which is the dominant UE, radicular Sx (dermatomal or sclerotomal)? *(see Appendices A and B)*

● Functional limitations

● SQ, if applicable: night pain, bilateral UE numbness/tingling, unexplained weight loss)

● Review of systems (cardiovascular, pulmonary, gastrointestinal)

# Objective Examination

I. Standing
   A. Observation
      1. Posture
      2. Abnormalities, deformities, atrophy
   B. AROM (note quality, scapulohumeral rhythm, pain, and common substitutions)
      1. Shoulder flex (165–180 deg)
      2. Shoulder ext (50–60 deg)
      3. Shoulder abd (170–180 deg)
      4. Shoulder horizontal abd and add
   C. PROM if lacking AROM in any motions
   D. Special tests (as applicable)
      1. Impingement: impingement relief test
II. Sitting
   A. R/O cervical pathology *(see Special Tests for the Cervical Spine in Chapter 2)*
   B. Observation
      1. Posture
      2. Abnormalities, deformities, atrophy
   C. AROM may also be assessed in sitting
   D. PROM if lacking AROM in any motions
   E. GMMT and myotomal screen
      1. Shoulder elevation/shrug (C3–C4)
      2. Shoulder abd (C5)
      3. Shoulder flex (C5–C7)
      4. Shoulder ext
      5. Elbow flex/wrist ext (C6)
      6. Elbow ext/wrist flex (C7)
      7. Thumb IP joint ext/finger flex (C8)
      8. Finger add (T1)
   F. MSRs, if applicable
      1. Biceps (C5–C6)
      2. Brachioradialis (C5–C6)

    3. Triceps (C7)
- G. Special tests (as applicable)
  1. Instability: anterior/posterior apprehension tests, relocation test, sulcus sign
  2. Biceps tendinitis/tendon instability: Yergason's, Speed's, Ludington's, and THL tests
  3. Impingement: painful arc test, Hawkin's impingement test, impingement relief test, Neer's impingement test
  4. Rotator cuff tear: drop-arm test, supraspinatus test (empty can test)
  5. Thoracic outlet syndrome: Adson's maneuver, costoclavicular syndrome test, or Halstead's maneuver; hyperabduction syndrome test
- H. Sensation: LT and 2-point discrimination
- I. Palpation
  1. Tendons of the rotator cuff
  2. Bicipital groove/biceps tendon
  3. Bony landmarks

III. Supine
- A. Special tests (as applicable)
  1. Impingement: impingement relief test (may be performed standing or supine)
  2. Joint play
     a. AP glide
     b. Long-axis distraction
     c. AP motions of the clavicle at the AC and SC joints

IV. Prone
- A. AROM
  1. Shoulder IR (70–80 deg)
  2. Shoulder ER (80–90 deg)
- B. GMMT
  1. Shoulder IR
  2. Shoulder ER

## SPECIAL TESTS FOR THE SHOULDER

| Test | Detects | Test Procedure | Positive Sign |
|------|---------|----------------|---------------|
| *Impingement Tests* | | | |
| Neer's impingement test[1, 2] | Impingement of long head of biceps tendon and/or supraspinatus tendon | Pt sitting or standing. Pt's arm is passively elevated through forward flex by examiner, forcing greater tubercle of humerus against acromion. | Reproduction of Pt's Sx |
| Hawkin's impingement test[3] | Impingement of inflamed supraspinatus tendon | Pt sitting or standing. Examiner forward flexes Pt's arm to 90 deg, and flexes Pt's elbow to 90 deg, then passively internally rotates shoulder, forcing supraspinatus tendon against coracoacromial ligament. | Reproduction of Pt's Sx |
| Painful arc[4] test | Pathology of subacromial origin (e.g., impingement, rotator cuff tendinitis) | Pt sitting or standing. Pt abducts arm in neutral position (no IR or ER). | Reproduction of Sx in a 60–120 deg arc. Pain stops or is dramatically reduced when humeral head glides inferiorly. "No pain → pain → no pain" |

| Impingement relief test[5] | Helps confirm Dx of impingement | Pt standing, performs active flex and abd 3–5 times while examiner records location of onset of painful arc range. Pt asked to give a subjective indication of amount of pain. Test is then repeated while examiner applies a gentle inferior or posteroinferior glide just before onset of recorded painful arc. Pt is then asked again to give a subjective indication of amount of pain. Test may be modified to a supine position | Outcomes and their interpretations are as follows:

*Complete relief of pain:* indicates that humeral head is capable of moving under subacromial arch without impinging. This indicates contractile tissue as primary cause and recommend a Rx regimen aimed at training contractile tissue to balance force couple and scapulohumeral rhythm (e.g., strengthening, proprioception, scapular stabilization).

*Partial relief of pain at same point in range of motion:* suggests that, in addition to contractile tissue weakness, noncontractile tissue is involved. Joint mobilization in addition to strengthening and re-education should be part of Rx regimen.

*No relief or reduction of pain:* indicates inability of humeral head to depress because of noncontractile tissue tightness. As part of treatment program, perform joint mobilization to restore accessory motions to achieve inferior and posteroinferior glide of humeral head. Inability to reduce pain by stretching and joint mobilization may indicate pathology other than impingement as source of pain. |

*Continued* ▶

# SPECIAL TESTS FOR THE SHOULDER Continued

| Test | Detects | Test Procedure | Positive Sign |
|------|---------|----------------|---------------|
| **Stability Tests** | | | |
| Anterior apprehension test[3] | Anterior instability | Pt sitting, standing, or supine. Examiner places Pt's shoulder in abd and ext rot (90 deg/90 deg). Then examiner applies an ext rot force. | Pt has look of alarm or apprehension and resists further motion. Pt may also have pain with this movement. |
| Relocation test[6] | Anterior instability | Pt supine. Same procedure as apprehension test. Upon finding a positive anterior apprehension test, maintain that position and apply a posterior force with one hand to the Pt's arm. | Pt's alarm or apprehension disappears, pain may be relieved, and further ext rot is allowed |
| Sulcus sign[3] | Inferior instability | Pt standing or sitting with arm by side and with shoulder muscles relaxed. Examiner grasps Pt's forearm below elbow and pulls distally/inferiorly. | Sulcus (gap) appears at glenohumeral joint Must compare with uninvolved shoulder |
| Posterior drawer sign[7] | Posterior instability | Pt supine. Examiner grasps Pt's proximal forearm with one hand and flexes elbow 120 deg. Then examiner positions Pt's shoulder in 80–120 deg abd and 20–30 deg flex. With other hand, examiner stabilizes Pt's scapula. As Pt's arm is internally rotated and flexed, examiner attempts to sublux humeral head with thumb. | Posterior displacement can be felt as thumb slides along lat aspect of coracoid process Pt may also have apprehension |

| Load-shift test[8] | Anterior, posterior, or multidirectional instability | Pt sitting. First, examiner places one hand over Pt's clavicle and scapula for stability. Then, grasping proximal arm near humeral head, examiner "loads" humeral head such that it is in a neutral position in glenoid fossa. Examiner then applies an anterior or posterior force, noting amount of translation and end-feel. | Excessive displacement anteriorly, posteriorly, or both compared with uninvolved shoulder |

## Miscellaneous Tests

| Cross-arm adduction test[8] | AC joint pathology | Pt sitting. Examiner horizontally adducts (passive) Pt's arm across chest wall. | Reproduction of Pt's Sx at AC joint |
| AC joint shear test[9] | AC joint lesion/DJD | Pt sitting. Examiner cups hands, with one hand on Pt's scapula and other hand over clavicle and then squeezes, causing a shear force at AC joint. | Reproduction of Pt's Sx at or excessive motion in AC joint |
| Yergason's test[10] | Unstable biceps tendon due to THL tear Could also detect biceps tenosynovitis | Pt sitting or standing. Pt's elbow flexed 90 deg, with arm at side of body. Examiner resists at wrist while Pt attempts to supinate a pronated forearm. | Localized reproduction of Pt's Sx in bicipital groove |
| Speed's test[3] | Bicipital tendinitis | Pt sitting or standing. Pt's shoulder is flexed with forearm supinated, and elbow is completely extended. Examiner palpates biceps tendon in bicipital groove and forces arm down in ext as Pt resists. | Reproduction of Pt's Sx localized to bicipital groove |

Continued ▶

| Test | Detects | Test Procedure | Positive Sign |
|------|---------|----------------|---------------|
| Ludington's test[11] | Rupture of long head of biceps tendon | Pt sitting or standing. Pt clasps both hands on top of head and interlocks fingers. Pt then simultaneously contracts and relaxes biceps muscles while examiner palpates biceps tendon proximally at bicipital groove. | Examiner feels tendon on uninvolved side but not on involved side during contraction of biceps muscle |
| Apley's scratch test[8] | Functional method of assessing shoulder in IR and ER | Pt performs combined IR with add in attempt to touch or "scratch" opposite scapula. Second motion involves combined ER with abd in attempt to place hand behind head and touch top of opposite shoulder. | Gives examiner an idea of functional capacity/AROM of Pt's shoulders<br><br>This is recorded by the anatomic landmark that Pt is able to reach and touch (e.g., to inferior angle of scapula) |
| Drop-arm test[9] | Rotator cuff tear (specifically, supraspinatus tendon) | Pt sitting or standing. Examiner passively abducts Pt's shoulder to 90 deg. Pt is then instructed to maintain arm in that position. Examiner then presses inferiorly on Pt's arm. | Arm drops suddenly to side because of weakness and/or pain |
| Supraspinatus test (empty can test)[6] | Torn supraspinatus muscle or tendon<br>Supraspinatus tendinitis<br>Neuropathy of suprascapular nerve | Pt sitting or standing. Pt in "empty can" position: 90-deg shoulder abd, 30-deg horizontal abd, and maximum IR. Examiner resists Pt's attempt to abduct. | Reproduction of Pt's Sx or weakness<br>Compare with uninvolved side |

| Test* | Detects | Test Procedure | Positive Sign |
|---|---|---|---|
| Adson's maneuver[12] | Entrapment in scalene triangle | Pt sitting. Examiner locates Pt's radial pulse. Pt then rotates head toward test shoulder and extends head/neck. Examiner then externally rotates and extends Pt's shoulder as Pt takes a deep breath and holds it. | Reproduction of pain and paresthesia in tested UE with diminished or absent pulse |
| Costoclavicular syndrome test[13] | Entrapment between 1st rib and clavicle | Pt sitting. Examiner palpates radial pulse and then draws Pt's shoulder down and back (depression and retraction). | Reproduction of pain and paresthesia in tested UE with diminished or absent pulse |
| Hyperabduction syndrome test[14] | Entrapment between coracoid process and pectoralis minor | Pt sitting. Examiner palpates radial pulse and hyperabducts Pt's arm so that Pt's arm is overhead. Pt takes a deep breath and holds it. | Reproduction of pain and paresthesia in tested UE with diminished or absent pulse |
| Halstead's maneuver[3] | Entrapment in scalene triangle | Pt sitting. Examiner palpates radial pulse. Pt then rotates head away from test shoulder and extends head/neck. Examiner then externally rotates and extends Pt's shoulder, applying downward traction as Pt takes a deep breath and holds it. | Reproduction of pain and paresthesia in tested UE with diminished or absent pulse |

*These tests detect subclavian artery and brachial plexus entrapment.

## TREATMENT OPTIONS FOR THE SHOULDER

| Special Condition | Hx/Symptoms | Signs/Objective Findings | Treatment Options |
|---|---|---|---|
| Impingement syndrome | Pain with overhead motion or when hand is placed behind back<br><br>Pain may refer down lat arm or anterior humerus | Positive painful arc<br><br>Positive Hawkin's impingement test<br><br>Positive Neer's impingement test<br><br>Must R/O cervical pathology<br><br>Check for instability that may be allowing impingement<br><br>Check for tight posterior and/or inferior capsule or muscle imbalance<br><br>Pt may have poor posture as a causative factor | *Acute:* relative rest, ice, NSAIDs<br><br>Gentle ROM (Codman's/pendulum, wand exercises)<br><br>*Subacute/chronic:* isometric shoulder flex/ext/IR/ER exercises progressing to isotonic (tubing or free weights) as Sx improve<br><br>May consider ultrasound to aid in healing/improve blood flow<br><br>Shoulder proprioception exercises<br><br>Closed chain shoulder stabilization (e.g., quadruped position and examiner applies perturbation to Pt)<br><br>Work on neuromuscular control of rotator cuff/shoulder girdle musculature<br><br>Scapular stabilization exercises (e.g., push-up with a plus, seated press-ups)<br><br>Posterior/inferior capsule stretch if indicated<br><br>Avoid overhead activities/work that aggravates Sx |

| Supraspinatus tendinitis | Pain with overhead motion or when hand is placed behind back<br><br>Pain may refer down lat arm or anterior humerus | Key finding is exquisite pain with resisted movement involving supraspinatus muscle (positive supraspinatus/empty can test)<br><br>R/O cervical pathology<br><br>Will also have positive impingement tests | *Acute:* relative rest, ice, NSAIDs<br><br>Gentle ROM (Codman's, wand exercises)<br><br>*Subacute/chronic:* isometric shoulder flex/ext/IR/ER exercises progressing to isotonic (tubing or free weights) as Sx improve<br><br>Supraspinatus-specific exercises<br><br>May consider ultrasound to aid in healing/improve blood flow<br><br>Closed chain shoulder stabilization (e.g., quadruped position and examiner applies perturbation to Pt)<br><br>Work on neuromuscular control of rotator cuff/shoulder girdle musculature<br><br>Scapular stabilization exercises (e.g., push-up with a plus, seated press-ups)<br><br>Posterior/inferior capsule stretching if indicated<br><br>Avoid overhead activities/work that aggravates Sx |
|---|---|---|---|

*Continued*

| Special Condition | Hx/Symptoms | Signs/Objective Findings | Treatment Options |
|---|---|---|---|
| Bicipital tendinitis | Pain over anterior shoulder<br><br>Does Pt perform repetitive curls/elbow flex against high resistance at work or recreation/weight lifting?<br><br>Pt may report "snapping" in region of bicipital groove | Exquisite tenderness to palpation over bicipital groove<br><br>May or may not have positive Yergason's or Speed's tests<br><br>May have exquisite pain with resisted horizontal add of shoulder that is in 90 deg ER<br><br>Check for posterior capsule tightness<br><br>R/O cervical pathology | *Acute:* Relative rest, ice, NSAIDs<br>Gentle ROM (Codman's, wand exercises)<br>Avoid AGG and initiate Pt education<br><br>*Subacute/chronic:* isometric shoulder flex/ext/IR/ER exercises progressing to isotonic (tubing or free weights) as Sx improve (avoid strenuous resistance in early phases)<br>IR stretch (towel/door stretch)<br>May consider ultrasound to aid in healing/improve blood flow or phonophoresis/iontophoresis for pain relief and to decrease inflammation<br>Shoulder proprioception exercises<br>Closed chain shoulder stabilization (e.g., quadruped position and examiner applies perturbation to Pt)<br>Work on neuromuscular control of rotator cuff/shoulder girdle musculature<br>Scapular stabilization exercises (e.g., push-up with a plus, seated press-ups) |

| Subacromial/subdeltoid bursitis | Pain at superior portion of glenohumeral joint | Marked restriction of shoulder flex and abd | *Acute:* relative rest, ice, NSAIDs, phonophoresis or iontophoresis |
| | Pain at night with difficulty sleeping | Tenderness to palpation over deltoid around acromion | *Subacute/chronic:* gentle prom (Codman's) progressing to AAROM (wand, pulley) |
| | Pain may radiate down arm | Distraction of glenohumeral joint inferiorly may relieve Sx | Isometric shoulder flex/ext/IR/ER exercises progressing to isotonic (tubing or free weights) as Sx improve |
| | | R/O cervical pathology | Joint mobilization |
| | | | May consider ultrasound |
| | | | Closed chain shoulder stabilization (e.g., quadruped position and examiner applies perturbation to Pt) |
| | | | Work on neuromuscular control of rotator cuff/shoulder girdle musculature |
| | | | Scapular stabilization exercises (e.g., push-up with a plus, seated press-ups) |
| | | | Pt education to avoid overhead activities/work |
| | | | Avoid overhead work/activities that aggravate Sx |

*Continued* ▶

## TREATMENT OPTIONS FOR THE SHOULDER *Continued*

| Special Condition | Hx/Symptoms | Signs/Objective Findings | Treatment Options |
|---|---|---|---|
| Anterior shoulder instability (after subluxation or dislocation) | Hx of acute traumatic abd-ER injury (fall on outstretched arm or grasp of arm during throwing motion) | Positive apprehension and/or relocation test<br><br>Positive load-shift test (with anterior translation) | *Acute*: radiographs to R/O Hill-Sach's or Bankhart lesion (if Pt being seen for the first time)<br><br>Protection (immobilization and Pt education to avoid shoulder ER with abd), ice, NSAIDs<br><br>Gentle ROM (Codman's, wand exercises) in painfree and apprehension-free range<br><br>*Subacute/chronic*: isometric shoulder flex/ext/IR/ER exercises progressing to isotonic (tubing or free weights) as Sx improve<br><br>Shoulder proprioception exercises<br><br>Closed chain shoulder stabilization (e.g., quadruped position and examiner applies perturbation to Pt)<br><br>Work on neuromuscular control of rotator cuff/shoulder girdle musculature<br><br>Scapular stabilization exercises (e.g., push-up with a plus, seated press-ups)<br><br>Pylometrics progressing to least stable position |

| Posterior instability (after subluxation or dislocation) | Hx of trauma | Positive posterior drawer sign<br>Positive load-shift test (with posterior translation) | Refer Pt to orthopedic surgeon if stability not improving<br><br>*Acute:* radiographs (if Pt being seen for first time)<br>Protection (immobilization and Pt education), ice, NSAIDs<br>Gentle ROM (Codman's, wand exercises) in painfree and apprehension-free range<br><br>*Subacute/chronic:* isometric shoulder flex/ext/IR/ER exercises progressing to isotonic (tubing or free weights) as Sx improve<br>Shoulder proprioception exercises<br>Closed chain shoulder stabilization (e.g., quadruped position and examiner applies perturbation to Pt)<br>Work on neuromuscular control of rotator cuff/shoulder girdle musculature<br>Scapular stabilization exercises (e.g., push-up with a plus, seated press-ups)<br>Pt education to avoid overhead activities/ work that aggravates Sx<br>Refer Pt to orthopedic surgeon if stability not improving |

*Continued* ▶

| Special Condition | Hx/Symptoms | Signs/Objective Findings | Treatment Options |
|---|---|---|---|
| Multidirectional instability | Pt C/O instability and may be able to demonstrate<br><br>Pt may have pain or impingement type Sx due to excessive movement/laxity of glenohumeral joint | Positive sulcus sign<br>Positive load-shift test (with both anterior and posterior translation) | *Acute:* relative rest, ice, NSAIDs<br><br>Gentle ROM (Codman's, wand exercises)<br><br>*Subacute/chronic:* isometric shoulder flex/ext/IR/ER exercises progressing to isotonic (tubing or free weights) as Sx improve<br><br>Shoulder proprioception exercises<br><br>Closed chain shoulder stabilization (e.g., quadruped position and examiner applies perturbation to Pt)<br><br>Work on neuromuscular control of rotator cuff/shoulder girdle musculature<br><br>Scapular stabilization exercises (e.g., push-up with a plus, seated press-ups)<br><br>Pt education to avoid activities/work that aggravates Sx or places Pt in an unstable position<br><br>If stability does not improve over several months of aggressive rehabilitation, refer Pt to orthopedic surgeon |

| | | | |
|---|---|---|---|
| Rotator cuff tear | May have Hx of FOOSH, throwing, or lifting injury<br>May be seen in older individuals as a result of degeneration of rotator cuff | Positive drop-arm test<br>Positive impingement signs<br>Positive painful arc test<br>Weakness of specific rotator cuff muscles<br>May observe abnormal scapulohumeral motion (i.e., scapular hiking before upward rot) | *Acute:* relative rest, ice, NSAIDs<br>Gentle ROM (Codman's exercises)<br>*Subacute/chronic:* isometric rotator cuff strengthening progressing to isotonic (tubing or free weights) as Sx improve<br>Shoulder proprioception exercises<br>Closed chain shoulder stabilization (e.g., quadruped position and examiner applies perturbation to Pt)<br>Work on neuromuscular control of rotator cuff/shoulder girdle musculature<br>Scapular stabilization exercises (e.g., push-up with a plus, seated press-ups)<br>If severity of tear warrants, surgical intervention/repair may be necessary |

*Continued* ▶

| Special Condition | Hx/Symptoms | Signs/Objective Findings | Treatment Options |
|---|---|---|---|
| AC joint separation | Hx of fall onto shoulder | Depending on severity of injury, Pt may or may not have a noticeable "step-off" from clavicle to acromion<br><br>Positive AC joint shear test<br><br>Positive cross-arm adduction test<br><br>Tenderness to palpation over involved AC joint | Immobilization in Kenny-Howard/AC joint sling (type I, 1 wk; type II, 2 wks; type III, IV, or V, until Sx subside)<br><br>Ice<br><br>Early ROM within limits of pain<br><br>Progress to general rotator cuff and shoulder strengthening as Sx subside<br><br>Rx of type III still controversial; some recommend surgical Rx, and others have obtained good results with nonoperative Rx. However, acute Rx of type III should be the same as for a type II injury. See the Cook, Dias, and Muller entries in the Bibliography for treatment options.<br><br>For type IV and V injuries, surgery is more of a consideration. See the Cook and Dias entries in the Bibliography for treatment options. |

| Adhesive capsulitis | Common for ages 40–60 yr | Restricted AROM in a clear capsular pattern (ER > abd > IR) | *Acute:* ice, NSAIDs, pain-relieving modalities in initial stages |
| | Several weeks' Hx of shoulder pain and restriction | | Codman's exercises for 2–3 min every 1–2 hr |
| | Pt may not be able to pull wallet from back pocket or fasten clothes that fasten in back | | *Subacute/chronic:* after pain subsides somewhat, begin stretching to increase ER, abd, and IR through wand exercises and joint mobilization |
| | | | Ultrasound to axilla to heat joint capsule before joint mobilization and AAROM/ stretches (remember to address glenohumeral, scapulothoracic, and AC joints) |
| Thoracic outlet syndrome | Sx include pain and paresthesia and possibly muscle weakness in shoulder, arm, and/or hand | Positive thoracic outlet syndrome tests | NSAIDs |
| | | Must differentiate from cervical pathology | Avoid AGG |
| | Very similar to cervical radiculitis/ radiculopathy | | Stretch appropriate structures causing Sx |
| | | | Neural stretch (scalenes, levator scapulae, pectoralis minor) |
| | | | Strengthen scapular stabilizers |

# References

1. Neer CS, Welsh RP: The shoulder in sports. Orthop Clin North Am 8:583–591, 1977.

2. Neer CS: Impingement lesions. Clin Orthop 173:70–77, 1983.

3. Hawkins RJ, Bokor DJ: Clinical evaluation of shoulder problems. In Rockwood CA, Matsen FA (eds): *The Shoulder.* Philadelphia, WB Saunders, 1990.

4. Kessell L, Watson M: The painful arc syndrome. J Bone Joint Surg Br 59:166–172, 1977.

5. Corso G: Impingement relief test: An adjunctive procedure to traditional assessment of shoulder impingement syndrome. J Orthop Sports Phys Ther 22:183–192, 1995.

6. Magee DJ: *Orthopedic Physical Assessment,* 3rd ed. Philadelphia, WB Saunders, 1997.

7. Gerber C, Ganz R: Clinical assessment of instability of the shoulder. J Bone Joint Surg Br 66:551–556, 1984.

8. Silliman JF, Hawkins RJ: Clinical examination of the shoulder complex. In Andrews JR, Wilk KE (eds): *The Athlete's Shoulder.* New York, Churchill Livingstone, 1994.

9. Davies GJ, Gould JA, Larson RL: Functional examination of the shoulder girdle. Phys Sports Med 9:82–104, 1981.

10. Yergason RM: Supination sign. J Bone Joint Surg Am 13:160, 1931.

11. Ludington NA: Rupture of the long head of the biceps flexor cubiti muscle. Ann Surg 77:358–363, 1923.

12. Adson AW, Coffey JR: Cervical rib: A method of anterior approach for relief of symptoms by division of the scalenus anticus. Ann Surg 85:839–857, 1927.

13. Falconer MA, Weddell G: Costoclavicular compression of the subclavian artery and vein. Lancet 2:539–544, 1943.

14. Wright IS: The neurovascular syndrome produced by hyperabduction of the arms. Am Heart J 29:1–19, 1945.

# Bibliography

Boissonnault WG, Janos SC: Dysfunction, evaluation, and treatment of the shoulder. In Donatelli R, Wooden MJ (eds): *Orthopaedic Physical Therapy.* New York, Churchill Livingstone, 1989.

Cook DA, Heiner JP: Acromioclavicular joint injuries: A review paper. Orthop Rev 19:510–516, 1990.

Dias JJ, Gregg PJ: Acromioclavicular joint injuries in sport: Recommendations for treatment. Sports Med 11:125–132, 1991.

Ellman H: Diagnosis and treatment of rotator cuff tears. Clin Orthop 254:64–74, 1990.

Hawkins RJ, Abrams JS: Impingement syndrome in the absence of rotator cuff tear (stages 1 and 2). Orthop Clin North Am 18:373–382, 1987.

Hertling D, Kessler RM: *Management of Common Musculoskeletal Disorders: Physical Therapy Principles and Methods,* 2nd ed. Philadelphia, JB Lippincott, 1990.

Itoi E, Tabata S: Conservative treatment of rotator cuff tears. Clin Orthop 275:165–173, 1992.

Karas SE: Thoracic outlet syndrome. Clin Sports Med 9:297–310, 1990.

Kisner C, Colby LA: *Therapeutic Exercise: Foundations and Techniques,* 2nd ed. Philadelphia, FA Davis, 1990.

Mulier T, Stuyck J, Fabry G: Conservative treatment of acromioclavicular dislocation: Evaluation of functional and radiological results after six years' follow-up. Acta Orthop Belg 59:255–262, 1993.

Neviaser RJ, Neviaser TJ: The frozen shoulder: Diagnosis and management. Clin Orthop 223:59–63, 1987.

Pink M, Jobe FW: Shoulder injuries in athletes. Orthopedics 11:39–47, 1991.

SHOULDER

3

# 4

# ELBOW

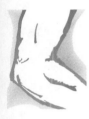

## Subjective Examination

- **Pt Hx (region specific):** dominant hand, radicular Sx (dermatomal or sclerotomal)? *(see Appendices A and B)*

- SQ (if applicable)

# Objective Examination

I. Standing
  A. Observation
    1. Posture
      a. Carrying angle for males (normal 5–10 deg valgus)
      b. Carrying angle for females (normal 15 deg valgus)
II. Sitting
  A. R/O cervical or shoulder pathology
  B. Observation
    1. Posture
    2. Atrophy or deformities
    3. Edema
  C. AROM
    1. Elbow flex (140–150 deg)
    2. Elbow ext (0 deg)
    3. Elbow pronation (70–80 deg)
    4. Elbow supination (80–90 deg)
  D. GMMT and myotomal screen
    1. Shoulder elevation/shrug (C3–C4)
    2. Shoulder abd (C5)
    3. Shoulder flex (C5–C7)
    4. Elbow flex/wrist ext (C6)
    5. Elbow ext/wrist flex (C7)
    6. Forearm pronation/supination
    7. Thumb IP joint ext/finger flex (C8)
    8. Finger add (T1)
  E. MSRs, if applicable
    1. Biceps (C5)
    2. Brachioradialis (C6)
    3. Triceps (C7)
  F. Special tests (as applicable)
    1. Instability: varus/valgus stress test

    2. Epicondylitis: tests for lateral and medial epicondylitis

    3. Nerve impingement/entrapment tests: Tinel's sign at the elbow, Wartenberg's sign, elbow flex test, test for pronator teres syndrome

G. Sensation: LT and 2-point discrimination

H. Palpation

    1. Soft tissue

    2. Bony landmarks

I. Joint play

    1. Radial and ulnar deviation (similar to valgus/varus testing)

    2. Ulnar distraction with the elbow in 90 deg flex

    3. AP glide of radius

4 ELBOW

# SPECIAL TESTS FOR THE ELBOW

| Test | Detects | Test Procedure | Positive Sign |
|------|---------|----------------|---------------|
| Varus stress test for elbow[1] | Rupture of RCL<br>Varus instability also associated with anterior radial head dislocation and annular ligament disruption | Pt's arm is stabilized with one of examiner's hands placed at elbow and other hand placed above Pt's wrist. Pt's humerus is placed in full IR, and elbow is slightly flexed (15–20 deg) as examiner applies varus force. | Laxity of involved elbow compared with uninvolved (note amount of laxity and end-feel) |
| Valgus stress test for elbow[1] | Rupture of UCL | Pt's arm is stabilized with one of examiner's hands placed at elbow and other hand placed above Pt's wrist. Pt's humerus is placed in full ER, and elbow is slightly flexed (15–20 deg) as examiner applies valgus force. | |
| Tests for lat epicondylitis[2] | | | |
| Method 1 | Lat epicondylitis | Examiner palpates lat epicondyle while pronating Pt's forearm and flexing Pt's wrist fully with ulnar deviation and extending Pt's elbow. | Pain/reproduction of Pt's Sx over lat humeral epicondyle |
| Method 2 | Lat epicondylitis | Examiner resists ext of middle finger distal to PIP joint, stressing extensor digitorum muscle and tendon. | Pain/reproduction of Pt's Sx over lat humeral epicondyle |

| Test | Identifies | Procedure | Positive finding |
|---|---|---|---|
| Tests for med epicondylitis[3] | Med epicondylitis | Examiner palpates med epicondyle, supinates Pt's forearm, and extends Pt's elbow and wrist fully with radial deviation. | Pain/reproduction of Pt's Sx over med humeral epicondyle |
| Tinel's sign (at elbow)[4] | Regeneration rate of sensory fibers of ulnar nerve | Examiner taps area of Pt's ulnar nerve in groove behind medial epicondyle. | Tingling sensation in ulnar nerve distribution of forearm and hand distal to point of tapping. Most distal point at which abnormal sensation is felt represents limit of nerve regeneration |
| Wartenberg's sign[5] | Ulnar neuritis (entrapment may be at elbow) | Pt sits with hand resting on table. Examiner passively spreads Pt's fingers and asks Pt to bring fingers together. | Inability to adduct 5th digit back to other fingers |
| Elbow flex test[6] | Cubital tunnel syndrome | Pt completely flexes elbow and holds it for 5 min. | Tingling/paresthesia in ulnar nerve distribution |
| Test for pronator teres syndrome[7] | Impingement of median nerve by pronator teres muscle | Pt sits with elbow flexed 90 deg. Examiner then attempts to supinate and extend Pt's elbow as Pt resists. | Tingling/paresthesia in median nerve distribution |

| Special Condition | Hx/Symptoms | Signs/Objective Findings | Treatment Options |
|---|---|---|---|
| UCL rupture | Hx of elbow dislocation, throwing injury, or chronic overloading, as in a throwing athlete | Positive valgus stress test of elbow<br>May or may not have tenderness over attachments of UCL | *Acute:* sling/immobilizer, ice, NSAIDs<br>Refer to orthopedic surgeon. Surgery may be considered<br><br>*Postop:* sling for a few days to 1 wk; maintain fingers/wrist AROM and grip strength<br>Cast brace (30–120 deg) for 4 wk; allow AROM within this ROM<br>Cast brace (0–120 deg) for 8 wk; allow AROM within this ROM and begin strengthening between 8–12 wk postop. Begin with isometric elbow flex/ext and wrist radial/ulnar deviation; progress to isotonic and isokinetic strengthening. In final stages, functional/return to sport activity should be initiated.<br>Resume throwing at 6 mo |

| Posterior elbow subluxation/dislocation | Hx of FOOSH injury with shoulder abducted or elbow in hyperextension | Radiograph confirms subluxation or dislocation<br><br>Dislocation normally requires relocation by medical personnel<br><br>Fx are common (beware!)<br><br>Be sure to perform a neurovascular assessment | Cast bracing times and ROM limitations may vary, but AROM within allowable restrictions noted above and progressive strengthening should progress as clinically reasonable and as patient tolerates.<br><br>*Acute:* ice, elevation, NSAIDs<br><br>If cleared by orthopedic surgeon (no Fx that require ORIF or prevent initiation of rehabilitation), may begin immediate motion<br><br>Maintain wrist and hand motion and strength<br><br>No instability: immediate unlimited motion without brace<br><br>Valgus instability: immediate unlimited motion in a cast brace with forearm fully pronated<br><br>Unstable in extension: immediate motion in cast brace that blocks full extension. Extension block may be gradually eliminated over 3–6 wk.<br><br>*Subacute/chronic:* begin isometric elbow flex/ext/pronation/supination and wrist radial and ulnar deviation. Progress to isotonic and isokinetic strengthening. |

*Continued*

47

**TREATMENT OPTIONS FOR THE ELBOW** *Continued*

| Special Condition | Hx/Symptoms | Signs/Objective Findings | Treatment Options |
|---|---|---|---|
| Lateral epicondylitis (tennis elbow) | Hx of overuse, heavy lifting, repetitive motions such as filing/keyboard work/tennis strokes (forceful pronation and supination) | Local tenderness to palpation over common wrist extensor origin (lat humeral epicondyle)<br><br>AGG: resisted wrist and middle finger ext<br><br>Positive lat epicondylitis tests<br><br>R/O C6 radiculitis or radiculopathy<br><br>R/O posterior interosseous nerve entrapment | *Acute:* decrease inflammation (ice, NSAIDs, phonophoresis or iontophoresis)<br><br>Relative rest<br><br>Epicondylar splint<br><br>*Subacute:* stretching wrist extensors and flexors<br><br>Transverse friction massage<br><br>Isometric strengthening for wrist flex/ext/radial and ulnar deviation (initially performed with elbow flexed, then progress to performing exercises with elbow extended)<br><br>*Chronic:* progress isometrics to isotonics<br><br>Strength and endurance training is focused primarily on wrist extensors<br><br>Pt education |

| Med epicondylitis (golfer's elbow) | Hx of high-intensity flex/pronation/gripping<br>Pain during activity that increases after activity | Local tenderness over med humeral epicondyle<br>AGG: PROM into full wrist ext and resisted isometric wrist flex with forearm pronation<br>Positive med epicondylitis tests | *Acute:* decrease inflammation (ice, NSAIDs, phonophoresis or iontophoresis)<br>Relative rest<br>Epicondylar splint<br>*Subacute:* stretching wrist flexors and extensors<br>Transverse friction massage<br>Isometric strengthening for wrist flex/ext/radial and ulnar deviation (initially performed with elbow flexed, then progress to performing exercises with elbow extended)<br>*Chronic:* progress isometrics to isotonics<br>Strength and endurance training is focused primarily on wrist flexors<br>Pt education |
| Olecranon bursitis | Hx of direct trauma to olecranon process | Swelling and erythema over olecranon process<br>Exquisite tenderness directly over olecranon process and swollen bursa | Ice, NSAIDs, phonophoresis or iontophoresis<br>May consider padding area for protection |

*Continued* ▶

**TREATMENT OPTIONS FOR THE ELBOW** *Continued*

| Special Condition | Hx/Symptoms | Signs/Objective Findings | Treatment Options |
|---|---|---|---|
| *Median Nerve Neuropathies* | | | |
| Compression at elbow | Paresthesia in thumb, index finger, and middle finger that is aggravated by activity<br>Weakness in muscles of forearm and hand innervated by median nerve | Loss/weakness of pronator teres muscle in addition to muscles of hand innervated by median nerve<br>R/O cervical pathology | Relative rest and NSAIDs<br>Splinting<br>Ultrasound and soft tissue mobilization<br>Phonophoresis or iontophoresis<br>Surgical decompression if conservative Rx fails |
| Pronator teres syndrome (median nerve compressed at pronator teres muscle) | Paresthesia in thumb, index finger, and middle finger that is aggravated by activity<br>Weakness in muscles of forearm and hand innervated by median nerve | Resisted forearm pronation and elbow flex reproduce Sx<br>Pronator teres muscle is spared when compression is at this level vs. elbow (i.e., MMT of pronator teres reveals no deficit)<br>R/O cervical pathology | Relative rest and splinting for 4–6 wk<br>NSAIDs<br>Decrease AGG<br>Ultrasound and soft tissue mobilization<br>Surgical decompression or steroid injections if conservative Rx fails |
| Anterior interosseous syndrome (branch of median nerve) | Hx of sudden severe forearm pain that resolves in a few hours<br>No reported loss of sensation | Weakness of FPL, PQ, and FDP<br>Pt unable to pinch tip to tip or flex DIP joints of digits 2 and 3 (positive pinch test)<br>Key is no loss of sensation<br>R/O cervical pathology | Relative rest and splinting for 4–6 wk<br>NSAIDs<br>Decrease AGG<br>Ultrasound and soft tissue mobilization<br>Surgical decompression or steroid injections if conservative Rx fails |

| | | | |
|---|---|---|---|
| Palmar cutaneous nerve compression | Pain over thenar eminence and proximal palm | Positive Tinel's sign at palmar median nerve site | Padding area of injury<br>Phonophoresis or iontophoresis<br>Local steroid injections |
| Carpal tunnel syndrome | See Special Tests for the Wrist and Hand table in Chapter 5 | | |
| Radial Nerve Neuropathies | | | |
| Radial tunnel syndrome (compression of radial nerve at elbow) | Pain over lat humeral epicondyle<br>Tenderness reported along line of radial nerve over radial head<br>Numbness in radial nerve distribution in hand | Resisted middle finger ext reproduces Sx more intensely than in lat epicondylitis<br>Resisted supination may also reproduce Sx<br>R/O cervical pathology and lat epicondylitis | Relative rest<br>Splinting<br>NSAIDs<br>Ultrasound and soft tissue mobilization<br>Phonophoresis or iontophoresis<br>Neural stretching |
| Superficial radial nerve compression | Numbness/decreased sensation over dorsoradial hand | Positive Tinel's sign over superficial branch of radial nerve<br>R/O cervical pathology | Remove tight wristwatch/band that may be causing compression.<br>Rest and splinting |
| Posterior interosseous nerve syndrome | Reported normal sensation (no paresthesia)<br>May have Hx of lat epicondylitis or increased use of supinator muscles | Reproduced Sx with forced wrist ext or digital compression when wrist is in flex<br>Wrist may deviate radially with wrist ext.<br>Pt unable to extend thumb or fingers at MCP joints<br>R/O cervical pathology<br>R/O lat epicondylitis | Relative rest<br>Splinting<br>NSAIDs<br>Address aspects of job/ADLs requiring increased use of supinator muscles<br>Surgical decompression if conservative Rx fails |

*Continued* ▼

| Special Condition | Hx/Symptoms | Signs/Objective Findings | Treatment Options |
|---|---|---|---|
| **Ulnar Nerve Neuropathies** | | | |
| Cubital tunnel syndrome (compression at elbow) | Paresthesia radiating to dorsal 4th and 5th digits | Positive elbow flex test<br>May or may not have benediction hand deformity<br>Positive Wartenberg's sign and Froment's sign<br>Nerve may sublux out of groove with elbow flex<br>R/O cervical pathology | Relative rest and avoid AGG<br>Instruct Pt to minimize elbow flex during ADLs<br>Modify work environment as necessary (e.g., pillow beneath elbow at desk, adjust height and angle of computer keyboard)<br>Splinting at night that allows no more than 30 deg elbow flex for 4–6 wk<br>Pressure pads over elbow<br>Phonophoresis or iontophoresis<br>Surgical decompression if conservative Rx fails |
| Ulnar nerve compression at wrist (at Guyon's tunnel/canal) | Burning sensation in digits 4 and 5<br>Sensory deficit of hypothenar palm and digits 4 and 5 | Weakness of all ulnar-innervated hand muscles<br>Positive Wartenberg's and Froment's signs<br>No motor loss of FCU and FDP to digits 4 and 5<br>Benediction hand deformity | Relative rest and avoid AGG<br>Splinting at night for 4–6 wk<br>Phonophoresis or iontophoresis<br>May require steroid and analgesic injection<br>Surgical decompression if conservative Rx fails |

# References

1. Regan WD, Morrey BF: The physical examination of the elbow. In Morrey BF (ed): *The Elbow and Its Disorders,* 2nd ed. Philadelphia, WB Saunders, 1993.
2. Lister G: *The Hand: Diagnosis and Indications,* 2nd ed. New York, Churchill Livingstone, 1984.
3. Hertling D, Kessler RM: *Management of Common Musculoskeletal Disorders: Physical Therapy Principles and Methods,* 2nd ed. Philadelphia, JB Lippincott, 1990.
4. Moldaver J: Tinel's sign: Its characteristics and significance. J Bone Joint Surg Am 60:412–413, 1978.
5. Hunter JM, Schneider LH, Mackin EJ, Callahan AD (eds): *Rehabilitation of the Hand: Surgery and Therapy,* 3rd ed. St. Louis, CV Mosby, 1990.
6. Magee DJ: *Orthopedic Physical Assessment,* 3rd ed. Philadelphia, WB Saunders, 1997.
7. Spinner M, Linscheid RL: Nerve entrapment syndromes. In Morrey BF (ed): *The Elbow and Its Disorders,* 2nd ed. Philadelphia, WB Saunders, 1993.

# Bibliography

Dellon AL, Hament W, Gittelshon A. Nonoperative management of cubital tunnel syndrome: An 8-year prospective study. Neurology 43:1673–1678, 1993.
Fess EE, Philips CA: *Hand Splinting: Principles and Methods,* 2nd ed. St. Louis, CV Mosby, 1987.
Galloway M, Demaio M, Mangine R: Rehabilitative techniques in the treatment of medial and lateral epicondylitis. Orthopedics 15:1089–1096, 1992.
Hertling D, Kessler RM: *Management of Common Musculoskeletal Disorders: Physical Therapy Principles and Methods,* 2nd ed. Philadelphia, JB Lippincott, 1990.
Kisner C, Colby LA: *Therapeutic Exercise: Foundations and Techniques,* 2nd ed. Philadelphia, FA Davis, 1990.
Linscheid RL, O'Driscoll SW: Elbow dislocations. In Morrey BF (ed): *The Elbow and Its Disorders,* 2nd ed. Philadelphia, WB Saunders, 1993.
Lister G: *The Hand: Diagnosis and Indications,* 2nd ed. New York, Churchill Livingstone, 1984.
Nirschl RP: Muscle and tendon trauma: Tennis elbow. In Morrey BF (ed): *The Elbow and Its Disorders,* 2nd ed. Philadelphia, WB Saunders, 1993.
O'Driscoll SW: Classification and spectrum of elbow instability: Recurrent instability. In Morrey BF (ed): *The Elbow and Its Disorders,* 2nd ed. Philadelphia, WB Saunders, 1993.

ELBOW

4

Schantz K, Riegels-Nielsen P: The anterior interosseous nerve syndrome. J Hand Surg Br 17:510–512, 1992.

Spinner M, Linscheid RL: Nerve entrapment syndromes. In Morrey BF (ed): *The Elbow and Its Disorders,* 2nd ed. Philadelphia, WB Saunders, 1993.

Yocum LA: The diagnosis and nonoperative treatment of elbow problems in the athlete. Clin Sports Med 8:439–451, 1989.

**5**

# WRIST AND HAND

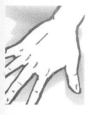

## Subjective Examination

▶ **Pt Hx (region specific):** dominant hand, functional limitations

▶ SQ (if applicable)

# Objective Examination

I. Sitting

A. R/O cervical pathology *(see Chapter 2),* shoulder and elbow involvement/pathology

B. Observation

   1. Posture
   2. Atrophy or deformities

C. AROM (note quality, pain)

   1. Wrist flex (70–80 deg)
   2. Wrist ext (65–80 deg)
   3. Wrist radial (15–25 deg) and ulnar deviation (30–40 deg)
   4. Digits flex/ext
   5. Opposition of digits

D. PROM (same motions if AROM limited)

E. GMMT and myotomal screen

   1. Elbow flex/wrist ext (C6)
   2. Elbow ext/wrist flex (C7)
   3. Finger flex (C8)
   4. Finger abd (T1)
   5. Grip strength with dynomometer

F. MSRs

   1. Biceps (C5)
   2. Brachioradialis (C6)
   3. Triceps (C7)

G. Special tests (as applicable)

   1. Carpal tunnel syndrome: Phalen's test, Tinel's sign at the wrist
   2. Ulnar nerve paralysis: Froment's sign
   3. Other tests for neuropathy: wrinkle (shrivel) test, sweat test, pinch test
   4. Vascular disorder/compromise: Allen's test
   5. Tenosynovitis/de Quervain's disease: Finkelstein's test

6. Contractures: Bunnel-Littler test, test for tight retinacular ligaments
7. Dislocation/instability: varus/valgus stress of digits maneuver, hyperabduction

H. Sensation: LT, 2-point discrimination, sharp/dull, hot/cold, monofilaments

I. Palpation
   1. Anatomic landmarks, especially the anatomic "snuff box"
   2. Soft tissue

J. Joint play
   1. AP glides
   2. Lat glides
   3. Radial and ulnar deviation
   4. Long-axis distraction

## SPECIAL TESTS FOR THE WRIST AND HAND

| Test | Detects | Test Procedure | Positive Sign |
|------|---------|----------------|---------------|
| **Nerve Lesions** | | | |
| Phalen's test (wrist flex test)[1, 2] | Carpal tunnel syndrome | Method 1: Pt has elbows on table with hands up and wrists flexed for 1 min<br>Method 2: Pt places dorsal surface of hands together, fully flexing wrists, and holds for 1 min | Tingling in thumb, index finger, middle finger, and lat half of ring finger |
| Tinel's sign at wrist[3] | Carpal tunnel syndrome<br>Can also be used to chart regeneration of lost sensory fibers | Examiner taps over carpal tunnel at wrist | Tapping causes tingling/paresthesia into thumb, index finger, and middle finger<br>Tingling is distal to point of tapping |
| Wrinkle (shrivel) test[4] | Denervation of fingers | Pt's fingers are placed in warm water for approx 30 min. Examiner then removes Pt's fingers and observes whether skin over pulp of fingers is wrinkled. | Failure of fingers to wrinkle; normal fingers wrinkle, but denervated fingers remain smooth |

| Test | Indication | Method | Positive finding |
|---|---|---|---|
| Sweat test (ninhydrin sweat test)[5, 6] | Denervation of fingers | Pt's hand is cleaned thoroughly and wiped with alcohol. Pt then waits 5–30 min and avoids contacting any other surface with fingers. Fingertips are then pressed with moderate pressure against good-quality bond paper that has not been touched. Fingers are held there for 15 sec and traced on the paper with a pencil. Paper is then sprayed with ninhydrin reagent to stain sweat areas purple. Allow 24 hours to dry. | No change in color, indicating lack of sweating |
| 2-point discrimination test (static)[1] | Decreased hand sensation | Using an object with 2 points separated by a known distance, apply light pressure to fingertips with 2 points simultaneously. | Inability to distinguish 2-point touch with more than 6-mm separation of points |
| Pinch test[7] | Compromised anterior interosseous nerve | Pt attempts to pinch using only tips of thumb and index finger or thumb and middle finger. | Pt unable to pinch tip-to-tip and has to resort to pulp-to-pulp pinch owing to weakness of FDP |
| Froment's sign[8] | Ulnar nerve paralysis | Pt attempts to grasp a piece of paper between thumb and index finger (add of thumb). Examiner then attempts to pull paper away. | Pt's terminal phalanx of thumb flexes because of paralysis/weakness of adductor pollicis |

*Continued* ▶

59

## SPECIAL TESTS FOR THE WRIST AND HAND *Continued*

| Test | Detects | Test Procedure | Positive Sign |
|------|---------|----------------|---------------|
| Wartenberg's sign[6, 9] | Ulnar nerve neuritis/paralysis | Pt sits with hand resting with palm flat on table. Examiner passively spreads Pt's fingers and asks Pt to bring fingers back together. | Inability to adduct the 5th digit to other fingers |
| **Miscellaneous Conditions** | | | |
| Finkelstein's test[10] | Tenosynovitis in thumb (APL and EPB) in de Quervain's disease | Pt makes fist with thumb held beneath flexed fingers. Examiner stabilizes Pt's forearm and ulnarly deviates Pt's wrist. | Reproduction of Pt's Sx over APL and EPB tendons |
| Bunnel-Littler test[11] | Differentiate tight intrinsic muscles from PIP joint capsular tightness | MCP joint held slightly extended while examiner moves PIP joint into flex if possible. | PIP joint unable to flex. If MCP joint is then flexed a few deg and PIP joint is able to flex, it was due to tight intrinsic muscles. If Pt unable to flex PIP joint in either position, it was due to tight joint capsule. |

| Test | Purpose | Procedure | Positive finding |
|---|---|---|---|
| Test for tight retinacular ligaments[11] | Differentiate tight retinacular ligaments from capsular tightness | PIP joint held in neutral position while examiner flexes DIP joint | Pt unable to flex DIP joint. If PIP joint is then flexed and DIP joint flexes easily, it was due to tight retinacular ligaments. If DIP joint unable to flex in either position, it was due to tight joint capsule. |
| Varus and valgus stress test[12] | Ligamentous instability of digit collateral ligaments<br>Useful in gamekeeper's/skier's thumb | Examiner grasps and stabilizes test finger.<br>Examiner then applies varus and valgus force at MCP, PIP, or DIP joint. | Laxity compared with uninvolved side |
| Allen's test[13] | Occlusion of radial or ulnar artery | Pt makes and relaxes fist several times and then squeezes fist tight to force blood out of palm. Examiner applies pressure over radial and ulnar arteries. Examiner then releases one artery. Hand should immediately flush red. Repeat for other artery. | Failure of hand to flush red immediately |

# TREATMENT OPTIONS FOR THE WRIST AND HAND

| Special Condition | Hx/Symptoms | Signs/Objective Findings | Treatment Options |
|---|---|---|---|
| Hypothenar hammer syndrome ("dunker's hand," injury to ulnar artery) | Hx of using palm of hand to push, pound, or twist<br><br>Pt reports coldness in fingers and palm<br><br>Pt reports tenderness over hypothenar eminence | Positive Allen's test<br><br>R/O other conditions such as thoracic outlet syndrome, Raynaud's disease, or Buerger's disease | *Acute:* rest from AGG<br><br>*Subacute/chronic:* modify activity with return to sport<br><br>If not improving, may require surgery |
| Scaphoid Fx | Hx of FOOSH injury<br><br>Pt points to pain in anatomic "snuff box" | Tenderness to palpation in anatomic "snuff box"<br><br>Limited/painful wrist motion<br><br>Distal pole of scaphoid may be tender on palmar surface<br><br>May be revealed on radiograph; not always able to tell on radiograph until osteonecrosis/avascular necrosis has begun | *Acute:* immobilization in short arm spica cast for a stable, nondisplaced Fx; surgery for displaced Fx<br><br>*Postop:* protective splinting, scar mobilization, edema prevention, AROM, isometric wrist/finger flex and ext wrist radial and ulnar deviation, progressing to isotonic PREs and functional strengthening activities, progressive hand weight-bearing activities (in later phases)<br><br>*Post casting:* same as after surgery, except no scar mobilization |

| | | | |
|---|---|---|---|
| Preiser's disease (osteonecrosis/ avascular necrosis of scaphoid) | Hx of FOOSH injury<br>Pt points to pain in anatomic "snuff box" | Tenderness to palpation in anatomic "snuff box"<br>Limited/painful wrist motion<br>Decreased grip strength<br>Radiograph shows "fat strap" in middle of scaphoid where bone resorption is occurring | Resection of scaphoid<br>Prosthetic scaphoid implant also possible<br>Vascularized bone graft surgery<br>*Postop:* protective splinting, scar mobilization, edema prevention, AROM, isometric wrist/finger flex and ext, wrist radial and ulnar deviation, progressing to isotonic PREs and functional strengthening activities, progressive hand weight-bearing activities (in later phases) |
| Kienböck's disease (osteonecrosis/ avascular necrosis of lunate) | Hx of FOOSH injury<br>Pt points to pain over area of lunate | Dorsal tenderness over lunate with localized swelling<br>Decreased grip strength<br>Radiograph becomes mottled, and lunate progressively deforms, eventually fusing to radius | Immobilization for 2–3 mo<br>May require resection of lunate and implantation of a prosthetic lunate<br>*Postop:* protective splinting, scar mobilization, edema reduction, AROM, isometric wrist/finger flex and ext, wrist radial and ulnar deviation, progressing to isotonic PREs and functional strengthening activities, progressive hand weight-bearing activities (in later phases) |
| Lunate dislocation | Trauma to hand in hit or fall | May be apparent in AP view as a wedge-shaped mass and in lat view in which capitate does not articulate with "cup" of lunate (which is rotated anteriorly out of its normal position) | Refer Pt to orthopedic surgeon |

*Continued*

**TREATMENT OPTIONS FOR THE WRIST AND HAND** *Continued*

| Special Condition | Hx/Symptoms | Signs/Objective Findings | Treatment Options |
|---|---|---|---|
| Gamekeeper's/skier's thumb | Hx of traumatic ext or abd of thumb<br><br>Pt points to pain over ulnar side of MCP joint | Instability of UCL of thumb<br><br>*Acute:* ulnar side of MCP joint tender, swollen<br><br>*Chronic:* UCL instability and functional difficulty; volar subluxation of proximal phalanx | Grade I: aggressive nonoperative rehabilitation<br><br>Grade II and III: surgery<br><br>Rehabilitation the same for nonoperative and postoperative treatment:<br><br>Thumb spica cast for 3 wk with MCP joint flexed 20–30 deg and IP joint left free to move to prevent scarring of extensor mechanism<br><br>Removable splint afterward for 3 more wk, gentle AROM<br><br>Continue to work on regaining full ROM; begin isometric strengthening, progressing to isotonics and functional strengthening activities |

| | | | |
|---|---|---|---|
| Rheumatoid arthritis in hand | Pt C/O pain and inflammation<br>Atraumatic | Positive RF on blood test<br>Must R/O septic joints<br>Tenosynovitis on dorsum of wrist where extensor tendons cross<br>Snapping or locking of tendon in sheath with movement<br>Contracture<br>Deformities include ulnar deviation of digits, swan neck, boutonniere, mallet finger<br>Muscle weakness<br>Instability | Rx based on stage<br>Control inflammation<br>Preserve integrity and maintain function of all tissues<br>Focus on joint systems, not isolated joints<br>Respect pain<br>Avoid deforming positions<br>Conserve energy<br>Maintain muscle strength and ROM<br>Pt education |
| Stenosing tenosynovitis of APL and EPB (de Quervain's disease) | Pt reports aching pain above radial styloid that radiates down hand and up arm<br>AGG: wrist and thumb motion | Positive Finkelstein's test<br>Tenderness and crepitus in first extensor compartment<br>R/O scaphoid Fx and carpometacarpal arthritis at thumb | *Acute:* ice, NSAIDs, phonophoresis or iontophoresis, may require cortisone/lidocaine injection, splint to relax APL and EPB (15-deg wrist ext, 40-deg carpometacarpal abd, 10 deg MP joint flex, and IP joint left free)<br>*Subacute:* isometrics for forearm and hand specific for pinch and grip strength<br>Gentle passive stretch<br>Intermittent release from splint<br>AROM to tolerance and progress to isotonic PREs to increase forearm, grip, and pinching strength |

*Continued*

| Special Condition | Hx/Symptoms | Signs/Objective Findings | Treatment Options |
|---|---|---|---|
| Carpal tunnel syndrome (compression of median nerve as it passes through carpal tunnel at wrist) | Insidious onset<br>Nocturnal burning pain in hand often reported<br>Pt reports loss of digital dexterity that interferes with ADLs | Positive Phalen's test<br>Positive Tinel's sign at wrist<br>Paresthesia in median nerve distribution of hand<br>At later stages, Pt may have thenar atrophy and/or ape hand deformity<br>R/O entrapment of median nerve at elbow or C6 radiculitis/radiculopathy | Pt education (avoid repetitive wrist flex-ext motions or prolonged wrist flex)<br>NSAIDs<br>Forearm splint to prevent constant wrist flex (splint holds wrist in neutral to 30-deg ext)<br>Tendon gliding exercises[14]<br>Wear splint 24 hr per day<br>Surgical decompression may be required if conservative Rx fails |
| Trigger thumb and trigger finger | Pt may describe "locking," "catching," or "snapping" of thumb or finger (ring or middle finger most common)<br>Pt may C/O Sx being worse on awakening and diminishing as Pt "limbers up" digit | Palpation of proximal flexor tendon may be painful<br>"Catching" is usually palpable as tendon slides through pulley | Refer Pt to orthopedic surgeon, who may consider a steroid injection<br>If problem persists, surgical release of tendon sheath may be performed |
| Ganglion cyst (at dorsoradial or volar radial wrist; can also occur at the flexor tendon sheath in the distal palm or dorsal DIP joint) | Pt reports painful lump/mass at wrist<br>Weight bearing such as push-ups aggravates Sx | Palpable, tender, solid mass at wrist | Splinting and relative rest<br>If unresolving, refer Pt to orthopedic surgeon for aspiration and possible surgical excision |

# References

1. American Society for Surgery of the Hand: *The Hand: Examination and Diagnosis,* 2nd ed. New York, Churchill Livingstone, 1983.

2. Lister G: *The Hand: Diagnosis and Indications,* 2nd ed. New York, Churchill Livingstone, 1984.

3. Moldaver J: Tinel's sign: Its characteristics and significance. J Bone Joint Surg Am 60:412–413, 1978.

4. O'Riain S: New and simple test of nerve function in hand. Br Med J 3:615–616, 1973.

5. Stromberg WB, McFarlane RM, Bell JL, et al: Injury of the median and ulnar nerves: 150 cases with an evaluation of Moberg's ninhydrin test. J Bone Joint Surg Am 43:717–730, 1961.

6. Hunter JM, Schneider LH, Mackin EJ, Callahan AD (eds): *Rehabilitation of the Hand: Surgery and Therapy,* 3rd ed. St. Louis, CV Mosby, 1990.

7. Wiens E, Lau SCK: The anterior interosseous nerve syndrome. Can J Surg 21:354–357, 1978.

8. Magee DJ: *Orthopedic Physical Assessment,* 3rd ed. Philadelphia, WB Saunders, 1997.

9. Blacker GJ, Lister GD, Kleinert HE: The abducted little finger in low ulnar palsy. J Hand Surg 1:190, 1976.

10. Finkelstein H: Stenosing tendovaginitis at the radial styloid process. J Bone Joint Surg Am 12:509–540, 1930.

11. Hoppenfeld S: *Physical Examination of the Spine and Extremities.* New York, Appleton-Century-Crofts, 1976.

12. Kahler DM, McCue FC: Metacarpophalangeal and proximal interphalangeal joint injuries of the hand, including the thumb. Clin Sports Med 11:57–75, 1992.

13. Allen EV: Thromboangitis obliterans: Methods of diagnosis of chronic occlusive arterial lesions distal to the wrist with illustrative cases. Am J Med Sci 178:237–244, 1929.

14. Baxter-Petralia PL: Therapist's management of carpal tunnel syndrome. In Hunter JM, Schneider LH, Mackin EJ, et al (eds): *Rehabilitation of the Hand: Surgery and Therapy.* St. Louis, CV Mosby, 1990.

# Bibliography

Amadio PC: Scaphoid fractures. Orthop Clin North Am 23:7–17, 1992.

American Society for Surgery of the Hand: *The Hand: Examination and Diagnosis,* 2nd ed. New York, Churchill Livingstone, 1983.

American Society for Surgery of the Hand: *The Hand: Primary Care of Common Problems,* 2nd ed. New York, Churchill Livingstone, 1990.

Bunt TJ, Malone JM, Moody M, et al: Frequency of vascular injury with blunt trauma-induced extremity injury. Am J Surg 160:226–228, 1990.

Cailliet R: *Hand Pain and Impairment,* 3rd ed. Philadelphia, FA Davis, 1982.

Fess EE, Philips CA: *Hand Splinting: Principles and Methods,* 2nd ed. St. Louis, CV Mosby, 1987.

Hertling D, Kessler RM: *Management of Common Musculoskeletal Disorders: Physical Therapy Principles and Methods,* 2nd ed. Philadelphia, JB Lippincott, 1990.

Kahler DM, McCue FC: Metacarpophalangeal and proximal interphalangeal joint injuries of the hand, including the thumb. Clin Sports Med 11:57–75, 1992.

Korkala OL, Kuokkanen HOM, Eerola MS: Compression-staple fixation for fractures, non-unions, and delayed unions of the carpal scaphoid. J Bone Joint Surg Am 74:423–426, 1992.

Lister G: *The Hand: Diagnosis and Indications,* 2nd ed. New York, Churchill Livingstone, 1984.

Newland CC: Gamekeeper's thumb. Orthop Clin North Am 23:41–48, 1992.

Philips CA: Rehabilitation of the patient with rheumatoid hand involvement. Phys Ther 69:1091–1098, 1989.

Rutherford RB: *Vascular Surgery,* 4th ed. Philadelphia, WB Saunders, 1995.

Spinner M, Spencer PS: Nerve compression lesions of the upper extremity: A clinical and experimental review. Clin Orthop 104:46–66, 1974.

Wadsworth LT: How to manage skier's thumb. Phys Sports Med 20:69–78, 1992.

Wilgis EFS, Yates AY: Wrist pain. In Nicholas JA, Hershman EB (eds): *The Upper Extremity in Sports Medicine.* St. Louis, CV Mosby, 1990.

# THORACIC SPINE

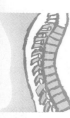

## Subjective Examination

▶ **Pt Hx (region specific):** Does coughing, sneezing, straining, or anything that increases intradiscal and intrathecal pressure aggravate the Sx? Sx with breathing?

▶ Does any particular posture aggravate Sx? Radicular Sx (dermatomal or sclerotomal)? *(see Appendices A and B)*

▶ SQ

▶ Review of systems (cardiovascular, gastrointestinal, pulmonary)

6 | THORACIC SPINE

# Objective Examination

I. Standing
   A. R/O lumbar spine pathology
   B. R/O nonmusculoskeletal abnormalities and tumors of the renal, pulmonary, cardiovascular, and gastrointestinal systems
   C. Observation
      1. Gait
      2. Posture (e.g., scoliosis, dowager's hump, kyphosis)
   D. AROM (note quality, pain) using methods such as fingertip to floor or down side of leg or an inclinometer
      1. Thoracic flex
      2. Thoracic ext
      3. Thoracic sidebending
   E. Myotomal screening
      1. Ankle PF (S1–S2): single leg-heel raise *(see Chapter 10)*

II. Sitting
   A. R/O cervical spine pathology
   B. Observation
      1. Function
         a. RFIS
         b. REIS
   C. AROM (note quality, pain) using methods such as inclinometer or estimation
      1. Thoracic flex
      2. Thoracic ext
      3. Thoracic sidebending
      4. Thoracic rot
   D. Myotomal screen*

*Myotomal screen and reflexes are commonly included in a lumbar spine examination and are included here because pathology in the thoracic spine can impact the results of these tests.

1. Shoulder elevation/shrug (C3–C4)
2. Shoulder abd (C5)
3. Elbow flex/wrist ext (C6)
4. Elbow ext/wrist flex (C7)
5. Thumb IP ext/finger flex (C8)
6. Finger add (T1)
7. Hip flex (L1–L4)
8. Knee ext (L2–L4)
9. Great toe ext (L5) (or supine)

E. MSR
1. Knee jerk (L3–L4)
2. Hamstring (L5)
3. Ankle jerk (S1)

F. Pathologic reflexes (if applicable*)
1. Babinski's
2. Clonus

G. Special tests (if applicable)
1. Dural irritation/nerve root involvement: slump test

H. Sensation (dermatomes) (*see Appendix A*)

III. Supine
A. Myotomal screen
1. Ankle DF (L4–S1)

B. Special tests (if applicable)
1. Dural/meningeal irritation—nerve root involvement: Brudzinski's sign, SLR (Lasègue's test), upper limb tension testing

IV. Sidelying
A. Myotomal screen
1. Ankle inv (L5–S1)

6 | THORACIC SPINE

---

*Myotomal screen and reflexes are commonly included in a lumbar spine examination and are included here because pathology in the thoracic spine can impact the results of these tests.

 2. Ankle ev (S1)
B. Palpation
 1. Palpate PPIVMs for gapping during flex/ext
V. Prone
A. Myotomal screen
 1. Knee flex (L4–S2)
B. Palpation (include ribs)
C. Joint play
 1. PACVP
 2. PAUVP
 3. Transverse pressure
 4. Costovertebral joints (rib springing)

# SPECIAL TESTS FOR THE THORACIC SPINE

| Test | Detects | Test Procedure | Positive Sign |
|------|---------|----------------|---------------|
| Slump test[1] | Increased tension in dura/meninges | Pt sitting on edge of table, with legs supported and hips in neutral and with hands behind back. Pt slumps into full thoracic and lumbar flex. Pt then flexes cervical spine maximally, and examiner maintains overpressure. Pt actively extends knee. Then examiner dorsiflexes Pt's foot. | Reproduction of Sx in back and radicular Sx |
| Brudzinski's sign[2] | Dural or meningeal irritation<br>Nerve root involvement | Pt supine. Pt passively flexes neck by pulling head to chest. | Reproduction of Sx in back, and Pt involuntarily flexes knees and hips to relieve back pain |

## TREATMENT OPTIONS FOR THE THORACIC SPINE

| Special Condition | Hx/Symptoms | Signs/Objective Findings | Treatment Options |
|---|---|---|---|
| Scheuermann's disease (juvenile kyphosis) | 12–18 yr old; M > F<br><br>Insidious onset of localized pain | Observable thoracic kyphosis<br><br>Radiographs show kyphosis and anterior wedging of vertebrae<br><br>May see tight hamstrings | Relative rest<br><br>Pt education/postural education<br><br>Back extensor strengthening<br><br>Hamstring stretching, if appropriate |
| Costovertebral joint dysfunction | Onset may be sudden or insidious (R/O rib Fx if sudden trauma)<br><br>Unilateral Sx over costovertebral joint<br><br>AGG: deep breath<br><br>Ease: maintained pressure on back, erect posture | Having Pt rotate to side of pain aggravates Sx<br><br>Palpation of joint/PA glides at costovertebral joint may reproduce Sx | Costovertebral joint mobilization<br><br>AROM exercises for thoracic spine<br><br>Postural education<br><br>Back extensor strengthening |
| Postural dysfunction | Insidious onset<br><br>Pt may describe occupation that places stress on thoracic spine (e.g., seamstress flexed over a sewing machine, computer operator without arm rests/support) | Pt demonstrates poor posture in sitting and/or standing<br><br>Localized tenderness | Postural education<br><br>Help Pt solve ergonomic problems at work/home that are contributing to problem<br><br>Back extensor strengthening, may consider scapular stabilization exercises and relaxation exercises such as shoulder rolls |

| Compression Fx | Osteoporotic individual | Diagnosis by radiograph | This applies only to anterior compression Fx with posterior structures intact (most common) |
| | Sharp pain with or without signs of nerve root compression | Flex is very painful | Spinal brace or support to help Pt maintain ext and prevent flex (e.g., CASH or Jewett brace, semirigid Taylor-type brace, dorsolumbar corset) |
| | Flex increases Sx | Single thoracic compression Fx characterized by a prominent spinous and wide interspinous space below prominent spinous process | Pt education about positions/activities that are beneficial or potentially harmful |
| | | Multiple thoracic compression Fxs characterized by progressive increase of kyphosis | Encourage positions/activities that promote spinal ext and avoid flex |
| | | | Teach Pt to roll to side when getting out of bed |
| | | | Use a good lumbar support when sitting |
| | | | Walking and other weight-bearing activities to help prevent further demineralization of bone |
| | | | Active and passive ext exercises as soon as Pt's pain is decreased to the point that these may be tolerated |

## References

1. Maitland GD: The slump test: Examination and treatment. Aust J Physiother 31:215, 1985.

2. Brudzinski J: A new sign of the lower extremities in meningitis of children (neck sign). Arch Neurol 21:217–218, 1969.

## Bibliography

Grieve GP: *Mobilisation of the Spine: Notes On Examination, Assessment, and Clinical Method,* 4th ed. New York, Churchill Livingstone, 1984.

Magarey ME: Examination of the cervical and thoracic spine. In Grant R (ed): *Physical Therapy of the Cervical and Thoracic Spine.* New York, Churchill Livingstone, 1994.

# 7

# LUMBAR SPINE

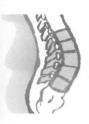

## Subjective Examination

▶ **Pt Hx (region specific):** Does coughing, sneezing, straining, or anything that increases intradiscal and intrathecal pressure aggravate the Sx?

▶ Nature of pain: radicular Sx (dermatomal or sclerotomal)? *(see Appendices A and B)*

▶ Specific postures that increase or decrease the pain

▶ SQ (night pain, bowel/bladder, saddle anesthesia, bilateral numbness and tingling in extremities)

▶ Review of systems (gastrointestinal, urinary, cardiovascular, endocrine, neurologic)

# Objective Examination

I. Standing
   A. Observation
      1. Gait
      2. Posture (e.g., lat shift, pelvic height/asymmetries, scoliosis, increased or decreased lumbar lordosis)
      3. Function
         a. Toe walking (S1–S2)
         b. Heel walking (L4–S1)
         c. RFIS/REIS
   B. R/O nonmusculoskeletal abnormalities and tumors of the kidney and prostate, UTI, AAA, and ulcers
   C. AROM (note quality, pain) using methods such as estimation, inclinometer, tape measure of excursion, and fingertips to floor or down side of leg
      1. Lumbar flex
      2. Lumbar ext
      3. Lumbar sidebending
      4. Lumbar rot
   D. Myotomal screen
      1. Ankle PF (S1–S2): single leg-heel raise *(see Chapter 10)*
   E. Special tests (if applicable)
      1. Quadrant test
II. Sitting
   A. Myotomal screen
      1. Hip flex (L1–L4)
      2. Knee ext (L2–L4)
      3. Great toe ext (L5) (or supine)
   B. MSR
      1. Knee jerk (L3–L4)

    2. Hamstring (L5)

    3. Ankle jerk (S1)

C. Pathologic reflexes

    1. Babinski's

    2. Clonus

D. Special tests (if applicable)

    1. Tripod sign

    2. Slump test

E. Sensation (dermatomes) *(see Appendix A)*

III. Supine

A. R/O hip pathology

B. Observation

    1. Function: RFIL

C. Myotomal screen

    1. Ankle DF (L4–S1)

D. Special tests (if applicable)

    1. Dural/meningeal irritation—nerve root involvement: Brudzinski's sign, SLR (Laségue's test)

    2. SI joint: SI joint gapping

    3. Leg length (apparent vs. true)

      a. Perform Wilson-Barstow maneuver first

    4. Sx magnification

      a. Hoover's test

      b. Waddell's signs[1]: superficial tenderness, rot and axial loading, distraction–SLR, regional sensation loss/weakness, overreaction

IV. Sidelying

A. Myotomal screen

    1. Ankle inv (L5–S1)

    2. Ankle ev (S1)

B. Special tests (if applicable)

    1. SI approximation

7 LUMBAR SPINE

V. Prone
- A. Observation
  1. Function: REIL
- B. Myotomal screen
  1. Knee flex (L4–S2)
- C. Special tests (if applicable)
  1. Prone knee-bending test
- D. Palpation
- E. Joint play
  1. PACVP
  2. PAUVP
  3. Transverse pressure

# SPECIAL TESTS FOR THE LUMBAR SPINE

| Test | Detects | Test Procedure | Positive Sign |
|------|---------|----------------|---------------|
| Quadrant tests[2] | Intervertebral narrowing/nerve root involvement (position of maximum intervertebral foramen narrowing) | Pt standing. Pt extends spine while examiner stands behind to control movement and apply overpressure in ext while Pt laterally flexes and rotates to the side of pain. | Sx reproduced down lower extremity to same side |
| Slump test[3] | Increased tension in dura/meninges | Pt sitting on edge of table with legs supported and hips in neutral and with hands behind back. Pt slumps into full thoracic and lumbar flex. Pt then flexes cervical spine maximally, and examiner maintains overpressure. Pt actively extends knee. Then examiner dorsiflexes Pt's foot. | Reproduction of Sx in back and radicular Sx |
| Brudzinski's sign[4] | Dural or meningeal irritation Nerve root involvement | Pt supine. Pt passively flexes neck by pulling head to chest. | Reproduction of Sx in back, and Pt involuntarily flexes knee and hips to relieve back pain |

*Continued*

81

| Test | Detects | Test Procedure | Positive Sign |
|---|---|---|---|
| SLR (Lasègue's test) with ankle DF variant[6–7] | Dural/meningeal irritation<br><br>Nerve root impingement due to disc protrusion or herniation | Pt supine. Examiner passively raises Pt's leg to where radicular Sx are reproduced. Leg is lowered slowly to where pain is relieved. Examiner then dorsiflexes Pt's foot. | Reproduction of radicular pain when leg is between 30 and 70 deg and pain reproduced again when foot is dorsiflexed |
| Tripod sign[8] | Dural/meningeal irritation<br><br>Nerve root impingement due to disc protrusion or herniation | Pt sits with both knees flexed 90 deg over edge of table. Examiner passively extends one knee. This can be performed during routine portion of examination after checking MSRs. | Pt extends trunk to relieve tension (or falls backward and supports body with UEs) |
| Babinski's reflex/sign[9] | Upper motor neuron lesion | Pt supine. Examiner runs pointed object along plantar aspect of Pt's foot and across metatarsal heads lat to med. | Pt involuntarily extends big toe and abducts (splays) other toes |
| Prone knee-bending test (femoral nerve test)[10] | L2-L3 nerve root lesion | Pt prone. Examiner hyperflexes Pt's knees bilaterally (heels to buttocks). This position is held 45–60 sec. | When knees return to 90 deg, Pt exhibits decreased MSRs and muscle weakness |
| Hoover's test[11, 12] | Symptom magnification or malingering | Pt supine. Examiner places one hand under each heel and Pt is asked to perform a SLR one leg at a time. | Pt fails to lift leg or examiner does not feel pressure under opposite heel |

| Test | Assesses | Procedure | Positive finding |
|---|---|---|---|
| SI joint gapping test[13] | Sprain of anterior SI ligaments | Pt supine. Examiner presses down and out on ASISs simultaneously. | Increased pain/reproduction of Sx in unilateral gluteal/posterior thigh |
| SI joint approximation test[13] | SI joint lesion dysfunction Sprain of posterior SI ligaments | Pt sidelying. Examiner presses down on iliac crest. | Reproduction of Pt's Sx, pressure or pain at SI joint (not at iliac crest or lumbar spine) |
| True leg length[14] | Leg length | Pt supine. Examiner measures ASIS to tip of med malleolus. Perform Wilson-Barstow maneuver first (see below). Relative length of tibia may be tested with Pt prone and knee flexed 90 deg. Examiner's thumbs placed on soles of feet. Note relative heights of thumbs. | Difference in measurements greater than 1–1.5 cm |
| Apparent leg length[15] | Lat pelvic tilt (could be AP rotated) | Pt supine. Distance from tip of xiphoid process or umbilicus to tip of med malleolus. | Difference in measurements |
| Wilson-Barstow maneuver[16] | Used for establishing symmetry before leg length measurement | Pt supine. Examiner stands at Pt's feet and palpates med malleoli with thumbs. Pt flexes knees and then pushes off with heels to lift pelvis from table. Pt returns pelvis to table and examiner passively extends Pt's knees and compares positions of malleoli. Tape measure can then be used to measure from ASIS to distal portion of med malleolus. | No positive sign. Is used to ensure symmetry before measuring leg length. |

## TREATMENT OPTIONS FOR THE LUMBAR SPINE

| Special Condition | Hx/Symptoms | Signs/Objective Findings | Treatment Options |
|---|---|---|---|
| Disc bulge or HNP | Most common at L4–L5 and L5–S1<br><br>Recurrent episodes usually show progression of Sx into extremity with each episode<br><br>AGG: any activity that increases intradiscal pressure (cough, sneeze, prolonged sitting)<br><br>Ease: any activity that decreases intradiscal pressure (supine lying with leg supported, stand better than sit) | Guarded/restricted movement<br><br>Loss of lumbar lordosis<br><br>Lat trunk shift<br><br>Positive SLR test/Lasègue's test<br><br>May or may not have objective neurologic signs (i.e., decreased MSRs, strength, and sensation in a specific dermatomal pattern)<br><br>Flex increases and may peripheralize Sx<br><br>Sustained or repeated ext decreases and/or may centralize Sx | *Acute:* attempt to correct lat shift if present and initiate McKenzie ext exercises (if they do not peripheralize Sx)[17]<br><br>Maintain lumbar lordosis and avoid positions that increase intradiscal pressure during healing<br><br>Elastic lumbosacral corset to reduce intradiscal pressure<br><br>Positioning for pain relief, lumbar roll<br><br>Moist heat or ice for anesthetic effect<br><br>Interferential electrical stimulation to help in pain modulation<br><br>Lumbar traction or positional traction<br><br>*Subacute/chronic:* progress to back strengthening/stabilization exercises<br><br>Aerobic training (walking, cycling, pool therapy) after Sx have centralized and decreased |

| | | | |
|---|---|---|---|
| Acute radiculitis/radiculopathy (nerve root becomes inflamed, causing compression that results in ischemia and loss of nerve root conduction [i.e., paresthesia, decreased MSRs, muscle weakness]) | Radicular Sx in dermatomal pattern (distal worse than proximal)<br>Constant, severe pain<br>AGG: cough, sneeze, forward flex | Pt looks ill<br>Movement severely limited (may stand with one knee flexed to decrease stretch on nerve root)<br>Positive tension signs (SLR test, slump test, or Brudzinski's sign)<br>Objective neurologic signs with radiculopathy (e.g., decreased MSRs, muscle weakness)<br>R/O piriformis syndrome | Pt education (posture, lifting, maintaining neutral position during ADLs)<br>Total management may be 6–12 wk<br>Refer Pt to orthopedic surgeon or neurosurgeon for progressive neurologic deficits<br><br>Requires caution<br>*Acute:* bed rest (1–2 d maximum), ice, Meds<br>Evaluate whether ext helps<br>Sustained lumbar traction<br>Positional traction<br>Monitor neurologic system each visit<br>Should see improvement in 7–10 d<br><br>*Subacute/chronic:* When ready, begin functional rehabilitation and educate Pt in proper body mechanics, protection, and strengthening of lumbosacral and abdominal muscles<br>If progressive neurologic deficits occurring, refer Pt to orthopedic surgeon or neurosurgeon. |

*Continued* ▶

85

| Special Condition | Hx/Symptoms | Signs/Objective Findings | Treatment Options |
|---|---|---|---|
| Lumbar spondylosis (DDD) | Central LBP; may radiate into buttocks<br><br>Does not radiate into extremity (but can if disc height is decreased to where it causes encroachment of intervertebral foramen)<br><br>Nature of pain: often a deep constant ache<br><br>AGG: activities that increase intradiscal pressure<br><br>Ease: positions that reduce pressure on disc and moist heat<br><br>AM stiffness that is eased with movement | Neurologic findings usually normal<br><br>Confirmed by decreased disc space on radiograph<br><br>Osteophytes/spurring at vertebral bodies may also be seen on radiographs<br><br>Limited lumbar ROM | General mobility exercise (e.g., supine lumbar rot) unless foraminal encroachment is present<br><br>Appropriate modality for pain modulation<br><br>Flexibility exercises<br><br>Initially, exercise in direction opposite of that which aggravates Sx (flex vs. ext)<br><br>May consider manual or mechanical traction<br><br>Joint mobilization techniques may be beneficial in presence of marked hypomobility<br><br>Aerobic training (e.g., pool, cycle, walk)<br><br>Elastic lumbosacral corset to reduce intradiscal pressure<br><br>Pt education, especially to avoid prolonged periods of sitting and other activities that increase intradiscal pressure |

| | | |
|---|---|---|
| Spondylolysis/spondylolisthesis; defect involving pars interarticularis, slippage of vertebral body occurring with spondylolisthesis | Most common site is L5–S1<br>Onset can usually be traced to vigorous activity or trauma involving forceful ext<br>Sx may be local or referred<br>Pt may have hyperlordosis<br>Ease: flex or sitting | Radiograph shows defect (Fx line across neck of "Scottie dog" in oblique/Scottie dog view)<br>Bone scan may confirm if this is suspected clinically but is unable to be determined by radiograph because it is in stress-reaction stage before Fx or it is a small or partial Fx<br>Exquisitely TTP with central PAIVMs over area of defect<br>Ext increases Sx, and flex decreases Sx | *Acute:* modalities, prescribe corset, and discuss with MD<br>Acute spondylolysis may heal with immobilization (bone scans helpful to distinguish between patients who have an established nonunion and those in whom healing is still progressing and who may therefore benefit from immobilization)[17]<br>*Subacute/chronic:* Flex exercises and abdominal strengthening<br>Back care and postural education<br>Avoid heavy labor/lifting and vigorous physical activity (e.g., flag football, soccer, wrestling)<br>If this is first time Pt has been seen for this, consider an orthopedic consultation<br>Fusion may be indicated in some Pts[18, 19] |
| Spinal stenosis | Male > female (2:1)<br>Hx of LBP for several years<br>Burning, numbness/tingling that radiates distally<br>May report B/B Sx and/or saddle anesthesia<br>AGG: prolonged standing and walking, lumbar extension | Must differentiate from Sx of vascular claudication<br>Radiographs may help confirm | Pt education<br>Flex exercises<br>Lumbar traction<br>Elastic lumbosacral corset<br>Carefully tailored aerobic exercise program (bike, walk, swim)<br>Refer Pt to orthopedic surgeon or neurosurgeon if Pt has progressive neurologic signs (B/B, saddle anesthesia, declining MSRs, progressive LE weakness) |

*Continued* ▶

## TREATMENT OPTIONS FOR THE LUMBAR SPINE *Continued*

| Special Condition | Hx/Symptoms | Signs/Objective Findings | Treatment Options |
|---|---|---|---|
| Apophyseal/facet joint impingement (impingement of synovial and capsular tissue between facet joint surfaces) | Sharp, unilateral, well-localized pain<br><br>Pt may report a sudden unguarded movement involving ext, sidebending, and/or rot | Pt has difficulty standing erect<br><br>Pt in a protective posture<br><br>Neurologic status is normal<br><br>TTP over involved apophyseal/facet-joint<br><br>Responds well to early mobilization or traction | *Acute:* rest, ice, and other pain-modulating modalities, lumbosacral corset<br><br>*Subacute/chronic:* progressive AROM, joint mobilization, traction, and/or flex exercises (to open up facets), back care education |
| Apophyseal/facet joint sprain | H/O moderate to severe trauma (e.g., twisting)<br><br>Sharp, unilateral, well-localized pain | Pt has difficulty standing erect<br><br>Pt in a protective posture<br><br>Neurologic status is normal<br><br>TTP over involved apophyseal/facet joint<br><br>Poor response to early mobilization or traction | Treated more conservatively than facet joint impingement because of likely effusion around joint<br><br>*Acute:* modalities, painfree movement, lumbosacral corset, and rest<br><br>*Subacute:* gradually increase mobility and may perform gentle mobilization<br><br>Guard against loss of normal lordosis from prolonged maintenance of protective posture |

| | | | |
|---|---|---|---|
| Ankylosing spondylitis (characterized by progressive joint sclerosis and ossification of ligaments first appearing in SI joints and spreading to lumbar and thoracic spine and ribs; severe cases can affect cervical spine and hips) | Pt typically 20–35 years old at time of onset<br><br>First noticed as vague LBP and stiffness that is worse at waking and eased with exercise<br><br>Intermittent Sx<br><br>Episodes may last weeks or months<br><br>Onset of each acute episode seems insidious, unrelated to exertion or activities | Loss of lumbar lordosis<br><br>Increasing rounding of thoracic and cervical spines<br><br>Laboratory tests reveal elevated sedimentation rates<br><br>Radiographs may be helpful in Dx only after several years, with earliest abnormalities seen in SI joints | Pt education is crucial. Encourage Pt to avoid heavy lifting work. Let Pt know that spine will eventually stiffen in a way that does not interfere with sedentary work and that pain is controllable.<br><br>Instruct Pt in positioning and postural exercises to resist gradual development of a flexed spine<br><br>Emphasize passive and active ext exercises<br><br>Pt should use lumbar roll when sitting to encourage ext<br><br>Encourage Pt to sleep on a firm mattress, to avoid lying flexed or in a fetal-type position, and to avoid using more than one pillow in supine position<br><br>Lumbar support, medication, and modalities may be helpful during acute episodes |

*Continued*

89

## TREATMENT OPTIONS FOR THE LUMBAR SPINE *Continued*

| Special Condition | Hx/Symptoms | Signs/Objective Findings | Treatment Options |
|---|---|---|---|
| Cauda equina syndrome (commonly caused by central disc bulge); a medical emergency | Saddle anesthesia<br>B/B Sx (urinary retention, loss of sphincter control)<br>Bilateral radicular Sx<br>Onset may be sudden or occur over a few hours to 1–2 d. | Lower motor neuron signs: progressive weakness, declining MSRs<br>Babinski's reflex/sign not present (i.e., cauda equina consists of lower motor neurons)<br>Gait abnormalities | Immediate referral to orthopedic surgeon or neurosurgeon |
| Malignant disease | Insidious onset<br>Localized pain<br>Unrelenting, continuous pain and getting worse<br>Night pain | Nothing relieves pain<br>Unexplained weight loss<br>Absence of pedicle on radiograph in AP view | Referral back to referring physician for further workup/referral |

# References

1. Waddell G, Main CJ, Morris EW, et al: Chronic low-back pain, psychologic distress, and illness behavior. Spine 9:209–213, 1984.

2. Corrigan B, Maitland GD: *Practical Orthopaedic Medicine.* Boston, Butterworths, 1985.

3. Maitland GD: The slump test: Examination and treatment. Aust J Physiother 31:215, 1985.

4. Brudzinski J: A new sign of the lower extremities in meningitis of children (neck sign). Arch Neurol 21:217–218, 1969.

5. Wilkins RH, Brody IA: Lasègue's sign. Arch Neurol 21:219–220, 1969.

6. Charnley J: Orthopedic signs in the diagnosis of disc protrusion with special reference to the straight-leg-raising test. Lancet 1:186–192, 1951.

7. Scham SM, Taylor TKF: Tension signs in lumbar disc prolapse. Clin Orthop 75:195–203, 1971.

8. American Orthopaedic Association: *Manual of Orthopaedic Surgery.* Chicago, American Orthopedic Association, 1972.

9. Dodd J, Kelly JP: Trigeminal system. In Kandel ER, Schwartz JH, Jessell TM (eds): *Principles of Neural Science,* 3rd ed. New York, Elsevier Science Publishing, 1991.

10. Herron LD, Pheasant HC: Prone knee-flexion provocative testing for lumbar disc protrusion. Spine 5:65–67, 1980.

11. Hoover CF: A new sign for the detection of malingering and functional paresis of the lower extremities. JAMA 51:746–747, 1908.

12. Arieff AJ, Tigay EL, Kurtz JF, et al: The Hoover sign: An objective-sign of pain and/or weakness in the back or lower extremities. Arch Neurol 5:673–678, 1961.

13. Magee DJ: *Orthopedic Physical Assessment,* 3rd ed. Philadelphia, WB Saunders, 1997.

14. Adams JC: *Outline of Orthopaedics,* 9th ed. London, Churchill Livingstone, 1968.

15. Hoppenfeld S: *Physical Examination of the Spine and Extremities.* Norwalk, CT, Appleton & Lange, 1976.

16. Woerman AL: Evaluation and treatment of dysfunction in the lumbar-pelvic-hip complex. In Donatelli R, Wooden MJ (eds): *Orthopaedic Physical Therapy.* New York, Churchill Livingstone, 1989.

17. McKenzie RA: *The Lumbar Spine: Mechanical Diagnosis and Therapy.* Wellington, New Zealand, Spinal Publications, 1991.

18. Hensinger RN: Current concepts review spondylolysis and spondylolisthesis in children and adolescents. J Bone Joint Surg Am 71:1098–1105, 1989.

19. Pedersen AK, Hagen R: Spondylolysis and

spondylolisthesis: Treatment by internal fixation and bone-grafting of the defect. J Bone Joint Surg Am 70:15–24, 1988.

## Bibliography

Grieve GP: *Common Vertebral Joint Problems.* New York, Churchill Livingstone, 1981.

Hertling D, Kessler RM: *Management of Common Musculoskeletal Disorders: Physical Therapy Principles and Methods,* 2nd ed. Philadelphia, JB Lippincott, 1990.

Kisner C, Colby LA: *Therapeutic Exercise: Foundations and Techniques,* 2nd ed. Philadelphia, FA Davis, 1990.

McKenzie RA: *The Lumbar Spine: Mechanical Diagnosis and Therapy.* Wellington, New Zealand, Spinal Publications, 1991.

Saunders HD, Saunders R: *Evaluation, Treatment and Prevention of Musculoskeletal Disorders: Spine,* 3rd ed, vol. 1. Chaska, MN, Educational Opportunities, 1993.

Schonstrom N: Lumbar spinal stenosis. In Twomey LT, Taylor JR (eds): *Physical Therapy of the Low Back.* New York, Churchill Livingstone, 1994.

Sinaki M, Lutness MP, Ilstrup DM, et al: Lumbar spondylolisthesis: Retrospective comparison and three-year follow-up of two conservative treatment programs. Arch Phys Med Rehabil 70:594–598, 1989.

# 8

# HIP

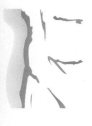

## Subjective Examination

▶ Pt Hx (region specific): H/O trauma, "snapping," "popping," or "grinding"

▶ SQ, if applicable

# Objective Examination

I. Standing
   A. R/O spine or SI joint pathology
   B. Observation
      1. Gait
      2. Posture
         a. Leg length (i.e., PSIS/ASIS level)
      3. Function (e.g., squat)
   C. Special tests
      1. Trendelenburg's test
II. Sitting
   A. AROM
      1. Hip ER (40–50 deg)
      2. Hip IR (35–45 deg)
   B. GMMT
      1. Hip flex (test sidelying if status poor or worse)
      2. Hip ER/IR (test supine if status poor or worse)
III. Supine
   A. R/O knee pathology
   B. Observation
   C. AROM
      1. Hip flex (120–130 deg)
      2. Hip abd (40–45 deg)
      3. Hip add (20–30 deg)
      4. Hamstring length
   D. Special tests (as applicable)
      1. DJD/hip joint pathology: Scouring test, Faber's test (vs. SI joint)
      2. Hip flexor length test: Thomas's test
      3. Piriformis syndrome: sign of the buttock
      4. Stress fracture: percussion test
      5. Leg length (apparent vs. true): perform

8

HIP

Wilson-Barstow maneuver first for improved symmetry

E. Sensation
   1. Dermatomes
   2. Nerve fields
F. Palpation
   1. Pubic tubercles/rami
   2. Inguinal ligament
   3. ASIS
   4. Iliac crest
   5. Greater trochanter
   6. Surrounding soft tissue/muscle
G. Joint play
   1. Long axis and lateral distraction
   2. Compression

IV. Sidelying
   A. GMMT
      1. Hip abd (test both supine if status poor or below)
      2. Hip add (test both supine if status poor or below)
   B. Special tests
      1. ITB: Ober's test

V. Prone
   A. AROM
      1. Hip ext (10–20 deg)
   B. GMMT
      1. Hip ext
   C. Special tests (as applicable)
      1. Anteversion: Craig's test
      2. Coxa vara or dislocation: Nélaton's line and Bryant's triangle
   D. Sensation
      1. Dermatomes
      2. Nerve fields

HIP

8

E. Palpation
1. PSIS
2. Iliac crest
3. Greater trochanter
4. Ischial tuberosity
5. Sciatic notch
6. Common hamstring tendon
7. SI joints
8. Surrounding soft tissue/muscle

# SPECIAL TESTS FOR THE HIP

| Test | Detects | Test Procedure | Positive Sign |
|------|---------|----------------|---------------|
| Thomas's test[1] | Hip flex contracture (tight iliopsoas, rectus femoris, TFL) | Pt supine with back flat on table and resting one leg off end of table with knee extended while flexing other hip, pulling knee to chest with hands, and holding | Straight leg rises off table |
| Rectus femoris tightness test[1] | Tight rectus femoris | Method 1: same as Thomas's test except tests LE with knee flexed | Method 1: flexed knee extends and is pulled up from table |
| | | Method 2 (Ely's test): Pt prone. Examiner passively flexes Pt's knee | Method 2: hip on same side spontaneously flexes |
| Ober's test[2] | Tight TFL or ITB | Sidelying with LE flexed at hip and knee to obliterate any lumbar lordosis. Affected knee is then held in 90 deg flex while pelvis is stabilized. Examiner passively abducts and pulls Pt's thigh/hip posteriorly until thigh is in line with body | LE remains abducted and does not fall to table |

*Continued*

# SPECIAL TESTS FOR THE HIP *Continued*

| Test | Detects | Test Procedure | Positive Sign |
|------|---------|----------------|---------------|
| Hamstring tightness test[3-6] | Tight hamstrings | *Method 1:* Pt supine with back flat on table. Examiner performs SLR test.<br><br>*Method 2* (modified active-knee-extension test): Pt supine and holds thigh so hip is in 90 deg flex. Pt then actively extends knee while examiner uses goniometer to measure angle formed by femur and tibia. | *Method 1:* straight leg being raised should raise at least 80 deg from table<br><br>*Method 2:* compare with opposite LE; although reported as a valid alternative to SLR test, no normative data exist for adults to author's knowledge |
| Sign of buttock[1] | Lesion in buttock and not in lumbar spine that is causing radicular pain | Pt supine. Examiner performs SLR test. If limitation exists on SLR, examiner flexes knee to see if more hip flex can occur. | Reproduction of radicular-type pain, even when knee is flexed |
| Scouring test[7] | Hip joint pathology (e.g., DJD, avascular necrosis) | Pt supine with hip flexed 90 deg. Examiner applies axial load and circumducts Pt's hip. | Exquisite pain reproduced in hip/groin and crepitus |
| Percussion test | Hip stress fracture | Pt supine. Examiner strikes heel. | Exquisite hip/groin pain |
| Faber's test (Patrick's test)[7] | Hip joint or SI joint problem | Pt supine. Examiner places Pt's foot of test LE on opposite knee. Test extremity is lowered in abd toward table. | Pain, muscle spasm, or limited motion<br>Positive findings with overpressure are indicative of SI dysfunction |

| Test | | | |
|---|---|---|---|
| Trendelenburg's test[7] | Stability of hip and ability of hip abductors to stabilize pelvis on femur | Pt stands on one leg | Pelvis on opposite side drops (unaffected side drops, and affected side shifts laterally) |
| Craig's test[1] | Measures femoral anteversion and indirectly measures hip stability | Pt prone with knee flexed 90 deg. Examiner rotates hip med and lat until greater trochanter is parallel with table or reaches limit of motion. Degree of anteversion then estimated based on angle of LE to vertical. | Anteversion greater than 20 deg, more common in females than males |
| Nélaton's line[8] | Dislocated hip, coxa vara | Pt prone. Imaginary line drawn from ischial tuberosity to ASIS of same side. Tip of trochanter should lie on or below this imaginary line. | Greater trochanter palpated well above this line |
| Bryant's triangle[8] | Dislocated hip, coxa vara | Pt supine. Imaginary line drawn from ASIS to table. Secondary line drawn through greater trochanter parallel to table and perpendicular to first line. Measure distance from secondary line to table. | Distance of secondary line from table greater on involved side than uninvolved side |

*Continued*

## SPECIAL TESTS FOR THE HIP *Continued*

| Test | Detects | Test Procedure | Positive Sign |
|------|---------|----------------|---------------|
| True leg length[9] | Leg length | Pt supine. Examiner measures ASIS to tip of med malleolus. Use Wilson-Barstow maneuver (see below). Relative length of tibia may be tested with Pt prone and knee flexed 90 deg. Thumbs placed on soles of feet. Note relative heights of thumbs | Difference in measurements greater than 1–1.5 cm |
| Apparent leg length[10] | Lateral pelvic tilt (could be AP rotated) | Pt supine. Examiner measures distance from tip of xyphoid process or umbilicus to med malleolus | Difference in measurements |
| Wilson-Barstow maneuver[11] | Used for symmetrization before leg length measurement | Pt supine. Examiner stands at Pt's feet and palpates med malleoli with thumbs. Pt flexes knees and then pushes off with heels to lift pelvis from table. Pt returns pelvis to table, and examiner passively extends Pt's knees and compares positions of malleoli. Tape measure can then be used to measure from ASIS to distal portion of med malleolus | No positive sign. This is used to ensure symmetry before measuring leg length |

| Special Condition | Hx/Symptoms | Signs/Objective Findings | Treatment Options |
|---|---|---|---|
| DJD | Groin or greater trochanter pain (especially with weight bearing), may also extend into lat or posterior thigh to knee<br><br>Insidious onset<br><br>Increased Sx with cold weather<br><br>AM stiffness and night ache | Increased Sx after activity (walking, running)<br><br>Increased Sx when hip in closed pack position, positive scouring or Faber's tests<br><br>ROM limitations in a capsular pattern | AROM<br><br>Maintain flexibility<br><br>Decrease stress on hip with activity (lose weight, exercise in a swimming pool, use assistive devices such as a cane)<br><br>Strengthen hip ext rotators and abductors |
| Trochanteric bursitis | May be insidious, or Pt may report specific event of feeling a "pop" as ITB snapped over greater trochanter<br><br>May have H/O direct blow to hip<br><br>Pain in lat hip that may refer along lat thigh to knee<br><br>Increased Sx with stairs, walking uphill, or sidelying on involved side | Tenderness to palpation directly over greater trochanter<br><br>May have positive Ober's test or Faber's test (or both) | *Acute:* relative rest, ice, NSAIDs, avoid AGG, phonophoresis/iontophoresis, ultrasound<br><br>*Subacute/chronic:* begin ITB stretching<br><br>If conservative Rx fails, refer Pt to orthopedic surgeon; orthopedic surgeon may inject or surgically excise bursa |
| Iliopectineal bursitis | Insidious onset<br><br>Pain in groin or femoral triangle | Tenderness to palpation in femoral triangle<br><br>Increased Sx with resisted hip flex and full passive hip ext<br><br>May have positive Faber's test | *Acute:* relative rest, ice, NSAIDs, phonophoresis, ultrasound<br><br>*Subacute/chronic:* hip flexor stretching |

*Continued* ▶

# TREATMENT OPTIONS FOR THE HIP *Continued*

| Special Condition | Hx/Symptoms | Signs/Objective Findings | Treatment Options |
|---|---|---|---|
| Piriformis syndrome | Pt may have Sx similar to radiculopathy, with pain (sharp/burning) in buttocks (unilateral) extending down LE<br><br>Pt may report that sitting or sitting in poorly cushioned chair reproduces Sx | Positive SLR, positive sign of the buttock, tenderness to palpation in sciatic notch<br><br>Increased Sx with hip ER or resisted ER | Ultrasound, piriformis stretching<br><br>Avoid AGG<br><br>If Sx fail to resolve/improve after 2–3 wk, may consider referral to orthopedic surgeon or pain clinic for injection |
| Legg-Calvé-Perthes disease | Groin, med thigh, and/or med knee pain (without knee pathology)<br><br>Sx in 3 to 8 year olds and in males most common | Antalgic gait<br><br>Pt has decreased ROM in abd, IR, and flex<br><br>Radiographs show flattened or resorbed femoral head | Refer Pt to orthopedic surgeon |
| Slipped capital femoral epiphysis | Insidious onset or may follow trauma<br><br>Sx in males during puberty and obese Pts most common<br><br>Hip &/or med thigh pain | Antalgic gait<br><br>Pt's hip automatically externally rotates when he/she flexes hip<br><br>Radiograph confirms | Refer Pt to orthopedic surgeon |

102

| Condition | Signs/Symptoms | Evaluation/Considerations | Treatment |
|---|---|---|---|
| Meralgia paresthetica (entrapment of lat femoral cutaneous nerve) | Pain/paresthesia in lat and anterior thigh<br>Pt may have had direct blow to iliac crest/ASIS<br>Overuse of abdominal muscles from sit-ups<br>Pt may wear tight belt or pants, causing Sx | R/O radiculopathy from back<br>Pt may be obese (putting pressure on nerve as it passes over ASIS)<br>Palpate along iliac crest/ASIS and inguinal ligament in attempt to reproduce Sx | Avoid AGG<br>Eventually subsides on own<br>May use ice for anesthetic benefit. Modalities and soft tissue mobilization if entrapment suspected rather than trauma |
| Pubic ramus stress Fx | Groin pain of insidious onset<br>Commonly occurs in short individual who overstrides to keep up with others when walking/running (e.g., military formation)<br>Aggravated by activity and relieved by rest | Antalgic gait<br>Tenderness to palpation on pubic ramus<br>Possibly adductor spasm<br>Bone scan consistent with stress Fx | Rest and crutches<br>After Sx subside, change training methods/schedule. Return to physical conditioning gradually |
| Femoral neck stress Fx | Groin, hip, and/or med thigh pain of insidious onset<br>Recent increase in physical activity/training<br>Aggravated by activity and relieved by rest | Positive percussion test<br>Bone scan consistent with stress Fx | Rest<br>Pt should be on crutches immediately because continued full weight bearing and physical activity may result in displaced femoral neck Fx and disruption of blood supply to femoral head |

## References

1. Magee DJ: *Orthopedic Physical Assessment,* 3rd ed. Philadelphia, WB Saunders, 1997.

2. Ober FR: The role of the iliotibial band and fascia lata as a factor in the causation of low-back disabilities and sciatica. J Bone Joint Surg Am 18:105–110, 1936.

3. Kendall FP, McCreary EK: *Muscles: Testing and Function,* 3rd ed. Philadelphia, Williams & Wilkins, 1983.

4. Gajdosik R, Lusin G: Hamstring muscle tightness: Reliability of an active-knee-extension test. Phys Ther 63:1085–1090, 1983.

5. Gajdosik RL, Rieck MA, Sullivan DK, Wightman SE: Comparison of four clinical tests for assessing hamstring muscle length. J Orthop Sports Phys Ther 18:614–618, 1993.

6. Cameron DM, Bohannon RW: Relationship between active knee extension and active straight leg raise test measurements. J Orthop Sports Phys Ther 17:257–260, 1993.

7. Maitland GD: *Peripheral Manipulation,* 3rd ed. Boston, Butterworth-Heinemann, 1991.

8. Beetham WP, Pollwy HF, Slocumb CH, Weaver WF: *Physical Examination of the Joints.* Philadelphia, WB Saunders, 1965.

9. Adams JC: *Outline of Orthopaedics,* 9th ed. London, Churchill Livingstone, 1968.

10. Hoppenfeld S: *Physical Examination of the Spine and Extremities.* Norwalk, CT, Appleton & Lange, 1976.

11. Woerman AL: Evaluation and treatment of dysfunction in the lumbar-pelvic-hip complex. In Donatelli R, Wooden MJ (eds): *Orthopaedic Physical Therapy.* New York, Churchill Livingstone, 1989.

## Bibliography

Barton PM: Piriformis syndrome: A rational approach to management. Pain 47:345–352, 1991.

Bunnell WP: Legg-Calve-Perthes disease. Pediatr Rev 7:299–304, 1986.

Hertling D, Kessler RM: *Management of Common Musculoskeletal Disorders: Physical Therapy Principles and Methods,* 2nd ed. Philadelphia, JB Lippincott, 1990.

Jankiewicz JJ, Hennrikus WL, Houkom JA: The appearance of the piriformis muscle syndrome in computed tomography and magnetic resonance imaging: A case report and review of the literature. Clin Orthop 262:205–209, 1991.

Kisner C, Colby LA: *Therapeutic Exercise: Foundations and Techniques,* 2nd ed. Philadelphia, FA Davis, 1990.
Schoenecker PL: Legg-Calve-Perthes disease: A review paper. Orthop Rev 15:561–574, 1986.

# 9

# KNEE

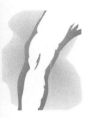

## Subjective Examination

▶ Pt Hx (region specific): Functional limitations, locking/popping/giving-way, swelling (if trauma, did it swell and how quickly)

▶ If traumatic, was there a "pop" at the time of the injury?

▶ Type of shoes (especially runners and running shoes): proper type, age of shoes, wear pattern

▶ SQ, if applicable

# Objective Examination

I. Standing

   A. R/O spine pathology

   B. Observation

      1. Gait

      2. Posture (e.g., genu recurvatum, genu valgum, genu varum)

      3. Function (e.g., squat, 1-leg hop)

II. Sitting

   A. GMMT

      1. Knee ext (test sidelying if status poor)

III. Supine

   A. R/O ankle or hip pathology

   B. Observation

      1. Posture (e.g., quadriceps angle, leg length differences, other alignment problems)

      2. Measure or grade effusion

   C. AROM

      1. Knee flex (135–145 deg)

      2. Knee ext (0 deg)

   D. Special tests (as applicable)

      1. Ligament: Lachman's test, varus and valgus tests at 0 and 30 deg, anterior and posterior drawer tests, pivot-shift test, flex-rot drawer test, ER-recurvatum test

      2. Meniscus: McMurray's test, bounce home test, joint line tenderness, Apley's grinding test

      3. Patellofemoral: apprehension test, grind test (Clarke's sign)

      4. ITB: Noble's compression test, Ober's test

      5. Plica: Swelling/effusion, tenderness over plica with palpation

      6. OCD: Wilson's test

   E. Sensation

9 | KNEE

    1. Dermatomes (*see Appendix A*)

    2. Nerve fields

  F. Palpation

    1. Specific anatomic landmarks/ligaments, including joint line

  G. Joint play

    1. AP and med/lat movement of tibia on the femur

    2. Superior/inferior and med/lat movement of the patella

    3. AP movement of the fibula on the tibia

IV. Prone

  A. GMMT

    1. Knee flex (test sidelying if status poor or below)

  B. Palpation

    1. Posterior knee complex

KNEE

9

## SPECIAL TESTS FOR THE KNEE

| Test | Detects | Test Procedure | Positive Sign |
|------|---------|----------------|---------------|
| Tests for Anterior Instability | | | |
| Lachman's test (modified)[1] | Compromised ACL (straight instability) | Pt supine. Examiner places knee and leg under Pt's thigh for support. Examiner holds proximal hand over knee, palpating joint line; distal hand is used to pull up on tibia just distal to joint. Pt's knee should be flexed 20–30 deg during test. | Excessive displacement of tibia compared with uninvolved knee |
| Anterior drawer test (also with tibial IR and ER)[2] | Compromised ACL (with IR and ER, may indicate anterolateral and anteromedial rotary instability, respectively) | Pt supine. Hip flexed 45 deg and knee flexed 90 deg with feet flat on table. Examiner stabilizes Pt's foot and pulls anteriorly on tibia. Also perform with tibia in IR and ER. Easy test to perform. | Excessive displacement of tibia compared with uninvolved knee |
| Pivot-shift test[3-6] | Anterolateral rotary instability (structures implicated as compromised are ACL, LCL, posterolateral capsule, the arcuate complex, and ITB) | Pt supine. Examiner grasps heel with opposite hand placed laterally on proximal tibia just distal to knee. Examiner applies valgus stress and internally rotates tibia as knee is moved from full ext to flex. | Tibia subluxes while femur externally rotates; then at 30–40 deg of flex, tibia suddenly jumps/reduces |

110

| Test | Instability/Structures | Procedure | Positive Finding |
|---|---|---|---|
| Flex-rot drawer test[7] | Anterolateral rotary instability (same structures implicated as in pivot-shift test) | Pt supine. Examiner holds leg (with foot under arm) and flexes Pt's knee 20–30 deg. While keeping tibia in neutral rotation, examiner then applies posterior drawer force on leg to cause reduced position. | Femur falls back posteriorly and externally rotates while examiner is holding Pt's leg and foot with knee flexed. When examiner then applies a posterior drawer force on Pt's leg, femur reduces and internally rotates. |
| Jerk test of Hughston[8] (reverse pivot-shift test) | Anterolateral rotary instability (same structures implicated as in pivot-shift test) | Pt supine. Examiner grasps foot with one hand and just distal to knee with other hand and applies valgus stress with IR of tibia and extends knee from 60 deg flex to 0 deg. | Sudden subluxation or "jerk" of tibial plateau at 20–30 deg knee flex |

### Tests for Posterior Instability

| Test | Instability/Structures | Procedure | Positive Finding |
|---|---|---|---|
| Posterior drawer test (also with tibial IR and ER)[9] | Compromised PCL (with tibia in IR and ER; may also indicate posteromedial and posterolateral rotary instability, respectively) | Pt supine with hip flexed 45 deg and knee flexed 90 deg with foot flat on table. Examiner stabilizes Pt's foot and pushes posteriorly on tibia. Also perform with tibial IR and ER. | Excessive tibial displacement compared with Pt's uninvolved knee |
| ER-recurvatum test[9] | Posterolateral rotary instability (structures involved include PCL, arcuate ligament, LCL, and posterolateral capsule) | Pt supine. Examiner grasps both of Pt's great toes and lifts feet from table (Pt told to relax quadriceps). | Knee assumes position of slight recurvatum, and tibia externally rotates. Involved knee/tibia appears to have tibial vara. |
| Valgus and varus stress tests at 0 deg knee ext[8] | Compromised PCL in addition to MCL or LCL | Pt supine with knee in full ext. Examiner holds Pt's foot under arm for support and places one hand along joint line and applies med and lat force. | Excessive med and/or lat gapping compared with Pt's uninvolved knee |

Continued ▶

| Test | Detects | Test Procedure | Positive Sign |
|------|---------|----------------|---------------|
| Sag sign[7] | Compromised PCL (straight instability) | Pt supine with hip flexed 45 deg, knees flexed 90 deg, and feet flat on table. Pt should relax muscles of LE. | Tibia sags posteriorly compared with uninvolved knee. |
| Godfrey's sign[7] | Compromised PCL (straight instability) | Pt supine. Examiner holds legs or places legs on something for support (e.g., stool) such that Pt's hips and knees are flexed 90 deg. Pt must relax LE muscles. | Tibia sags posteriorly compared with uninvolved knee, similar to SAG sign, above |
| *Tests for Medial and Lateral Instability* | | | |
| Valgus stress test (at 0 and 30 deg)[8] | Torn MCL. Straight instability with knee fully extended also indicates torn PCL. | Pt supine. Examiner holds Pt's foot under arm for support and places one hand along joint line and applies inward (med) pressure with opposite hand. | Excessive med gapping compared with Pt's uninvolved knee |
| Varus stress test (at 0 and 30 deg)[8] | Torn LCL. Straight instability with knee fully extended also indicates torn PCL. | Pt supine. Examiner holds Pt's foot under arm for support and places one hand along joint line and applies outward (lat) pressure with opposite hand. | Excessive lat gapping compared with Pt's uninvolved knee |

## Tests for Meniscal Tears

| Test | Clinical Condition | Procedure | Positive Finding |
|---|---|---|---|
| McMurray's test[10,11] | Posterior meniscal tears | Pt supine. Examiner grasps heel with one hand and places other hand on knee, palpating joint line (med and lat). Examiner applies full IR, then ER, as examiner takes knee from full flex to 90 deg. | Palpable click/pop and pain along joint line |
| Apley's grinding test[12] | Torn meniscus | Pt prone. Leg flexed 90 deg. Examiner leans hard on heel to compress menisci, rotating tibia internally and externally. | Eliciting exquisite joint line pain: med pain = med meniscus, lat pain = lat meniscus |
| Bounce home test[13] | Torn meniscus or loose body in knee | Pt supine. Examiner holds tibia with both hands and fully flexes Pt's knee, then allows knee to passively extend. | Failure of knee to reach full ext and exhibiting elastic resistance to further ext |

## Miscellaneous Tests

| Test | Clinical Condition | Procedure | Positive Finding |
|---|---|---|---|
| Apprehension test[14] | Patellar subluxation or hypermobility (with propensity for subluxation or dislocation) | Pt sitting with knees fully extended on table or supine. Examiner applies med and lat force to patella. | Pt feels like patella may dislocate and shows apprehension |
| Grind test (Clarke's sign)[7] | Patellofemoral joint disorder (e.g., DJD, patellofemoral pain syndrome, chondromalacia patellae) | Examiner places web space of hand just superior to patella while applying pressure. Pt gently and gradually contracts quadriceps. | Pain in patellofemoral joint. (However, many Pts feel pain with this test.) |

*Continued* ▶

| Test | Detects | Test Procedure | Positive Sign |
|------|---------|----------------|---------------|
| Wilson's test[7] | OCD | Pt sitting with knee flexed over edge of table. Pt then actively extends knee while examiner internally rotates Pt's tibia (IR of tibia puts tibial spine against lat surface of med femoral condyle, a classic site of OCD). | Exquisite pain with this motion at approx 30 deg of flex, then no pain when tibia is externally rotated |
| Noble's compression test[15] | ITB friction syndrome existing at lat knee | Pt supine. Knee flexed 90 deg with hip flexed. Examiner applies pressure with thumb over ITB just proximal to lat femoral epicondyle, and Pt actively extends knee. | Exquisite pain over distal ITB at point of pressure 30 deg before full knee ext |
| Ober's test[16] | Tight TFL or ITB | Pt sidelying with LE flexed at hip and knee to obliterate any lumbar lordosis. Affected knee is then held in 90 deg of flex while pelvis is stabilized. Examiner passively abducts and extends Pt's thigh/hip until thigh is in line with body. | LE remains abducted and does not fall to table. |

## TREATMENT OPTIONS FOR THE KNEE

| Special Condition | Hx/Symptoms | Signs/Objective Findings | Treatment Options |
|---|---|---|---|
| ACL deficiency/tear | H/O valgus or hyperextension force to knee if contact injury<br>H/O quick stop, landing with knee fully extended, or sharp cut with noncontact injury<br>H/O audible "pop"<br>Immediate effusion | Positive anterior instability tests<br>Pt holds knee in slight flex and unable to bear weight on involved LE<br>Rarely an isolated injury; look for Sx of MCL and meniscal injury | *Acute:* relative rest, ice, elevation, NSAIDs to reduce effusion; brace and crutches<br>*Subacute:* Quadriceps and hamstring sets, SLR, hip ADD/ABD<br>Progress to isotonic, closed-chain, and isokinetic hamstring and quadriceps strengthening; plyometrics; functional exercises for return to sport.<br>Pt also needs referral to orthopedic surgeon<br>Most facilities have their own postsurgical protocol if surgery is required |
| MCL deficiency/tear | H/O valgus force to knee through contact or noncontact injury<br>Pt C/O med knee pain | Pt may or may not have positive valgus stress test at 30 deg, depending on severity<br>Tenderness over MCL and/or attachments | *Acute:* relative rest, ice, elevation, NSAIDs; brace and crutches<br>*Subacute:* Quadriceps and hamstring sets, SLR, hip add/abd, stationary bike<br>When Pt has 90 deg knee flex, begin isotonic PREs and closed-chain exercises for quadriceps and hamstring strengthening<br>When Pt has full knee ROM, begin functional running program |

*Continued* ▶

115

**TREATMENT OPTIONS FOR THE KNEE** *Continued*

| Special Condition | Hx/Symptoms | Signs/Objective Findings | Treatment Options |
|---|---|---|---|
| LCL deficiency/tear | H/O varus force to knee through contact or noncontact injury<br><br>Pt C/O lat knee pain | Pt may or may not have positive varus stress test at 30 deg, depending on severity<br><br>Tenderness over LCL and/or attachments<br><br>Differentiate from ITB friction syndrome (H/O overuse and/or positive Noble's compression test) | *Acute:* relative rest, ice, elevation, NSAIDs; brace and crutches<br><br>*Subacute:* Quadriceps and hamstring sets, SLR, hip add/abd, stationary bike<br><br>Progress to isotonic, PREs, and closed-chain exercises for quadriceps and hamstring strengthening<br><br>As Pt continues to improve, progress to functional running program and return to sport activities |
| ITB friction syndrome | H/O increase in running distance, intensity, duration, or frequency<br><br>Pain over lat knee | Positive Noble's compression test, positive Ober's test (most likely)<br><br>Tenderness with palpation around lat femoral epicondyle<br><br>Differentiate from LCL sprain/tear | Relative rest, ice, NSAIDs, phonophoresis/iontophoresis<br><br>ITB stretching<br><br>Attempt to correct contributing biomechanical factors<br><br>Pt education to avoid future training errors and ensure that running shoes are not worn out |

| | | |
|---|---|---|
| Patellofemoral pain (PFPS, RPPS, PFJS) | Pain around/under "kneecap"<br>Pt may describe crepitus beneath/around "kneecap"<br>Ascending stairs especially aggravates Sx<br>Prolonged sitting with knees flexed may aggravate Sx (movie-goer's sign) | Positive or negative grind test (Clarke's sign)<br>Tender with palpation beneath med and/or lat borders<br>Pain with compression of patella | *Acute:* relative rest, ice, NSAIDs initially; may consider patellar taping away from painful patellar margin<br>Check for abnormal biomechanics (pes planus, patellar tilt or hypo/hypermobility, excessive Q-angle, tight hamstrings/calf/ITB)<br>*Subacute:* quadriceps sets, SLR, hamstring/calf/ITB stretching; progress to short-arc quadriceps and one-quarter wall squats/slides, standing quadriceps sets, pain free leg press<br>Also may consider backward walking on treadmill to strengthen quadriceps without increasing patellofemoral joint compressive forces |
| Patellar subluxation/dislocation | H/O valgus force and/or rot force to knee<br>Med knee tenderness due to tearing of med patellar retinacular fibers<br>More common in females | Positive apprehension test<br>Patellar hypermobility, effusion | *Acute:* relative rest, ice, elevation, brace<br>*Subacute:* quadriceps sets, SLR, hip add<br>Progress to short-arc quadriceps, one-quarter wall squats, forward and lat step-ups (focus on VMO) backward walking on treadmill, functional training |

*Continued*

# TREATMENT OPTIONS FOR THE KNEE *Continued*

| Special Condition | Hx/Symptoms | Signs/Objective Findings | Treatment Options |
|---|---|---|---|
| Symptomatic plica | Pain over med or lat femoral epicondyle<br><br>Pain with activity<br><br>Snapping sensation | Tender band or palpable cord from patella across med or lat femoral condyle<br><br>Must differentiate from patellofemoral pain<br><br>Arthroscopy is "gold standard" for Dx | *Acute:* relative rest, NSAIDs, ice, phonophoresis/iontophoresis<br><br>*Subacute/chronic:* quadriceps strengthening and stretching<br><br>If unresolving, may require arthroscopic excision by orthopedic surgeon |
| Patellar tendinitis ("jumper's knee") | H/O running, jumping, kicking, or climbing<br><br>Sx located along patellar tendon | Tenderness with palpation at inferior pole of patella or along patellar tendon, including insertion at the tibial tubercle<br><br>Single-leg hopping increases specific Sx at tendon<br><br>Possibly crepitus in tendon with ROM | *Acute:* relative rest, ice, NSAIDs, phonophoresis/iontophoresis<br><br>Pt education on how to avoid future incidences (proper training)<br><br>*Subacute/chronic:* progress back to full function |

| | | | |
|---|---|---|---|
| Osgood-Schlatter disease/syndrome | Occurs in children around puberty<br>Pain at tibial tubercle | Exostosis causing enlarged tibial tubercle<br>Point tenderness at tibial tubercle<br>Increased Sx with activity and decreased Sx with rest<br>Increased tibial tubercle pain with resisted knee ext | Relative rest<br>Decrease athletic activity (usually resolves as skeletal system matures, but enlarged tibial tubercle remains)<br>Quadriceps stretching and strengthening (e.g., sets, SLR) as pain subsides |
| Prepatellar bursitis | H/O acute blow to patella<br>Painful focal swelling | Tenderness and swelling directly on patella | Relative rest, ice, compression, NSAIDs, phonophoresis/iontophoresis<br>Stubborn cases may require aspiration by orthopedic physician or excision |
| Pes anserinus bursitis | Possible H/O blow to med proximal tibia (knee) or overuse<br>Painful area over tendons forming pes anserinus | Tenderness and swelling directly over region of tendons forming pes anserinus<br>Resisted hip add; may increase Sx<br>Be careful to R/O MCL sprain/tear or med meniscal tear | Relative rest, ice, NSAIDs, phonophoresis/iontophoresis<br>Stubborn cases may require injection, aspiration, or excision by orthopedic physician |

# References

1. Jonson T, Although B, Peterson L, Renstrom P: Clinical diagnosis of ruptures of the anterior cruciate ligament: A comparative study of the Lachman test and the anterior drawer sign. Am J Sports Med 10:100–102, 1982.

2. Weatherwax RJ: Anterior drawer sign. Clin Orthop 154:318–319, 1981.

3. Fetto JF, Marshall JL: Injury to the anterior cruciate ligament producing the pivot-shift sign: An experimental study on cadaver specimens. J Bone Joint Surg Am 61:710–713, 1979.

4. Galway HR, MacIntosh DL: The lateral pivot shift: A symptom and sign of anterior cruciate ligament insufficiency. Clin Orthop 147:45–50, 1980.

5. Tamea CD, Henning CE: Pathomechanics of the pivot shift maneuver: An instant center of analysis. Am J Sports Med 9:31–37, 1981.

6. Katz JW, Fingeroth RJ: The diagnostic accuracy of ruptures of the anterior cruciate ligament comparing the Lachman test, the anterior drawer sign, and the pivot-shift test in acute and chronic knee injuries. Am J Sports Med 14:88–91, 1986.

7. Magee DJ: *Orthopedic Physical Assessment,* 3rd ed. Philadelphia, WB Saunders, 1997.

8. Muller W: *The Knee: Form, Function, and Ligament Reconstruction.* New York, Springer-Verlag, 1983.

9. Hughston JC, Norwood LA: The posterolateral drawer test and external rotation recurvatum test for posterolateral rotary instability of the knee. Clin Orthop 147:82–87, 1980.

10. McMurray TP: The semilunar cartilage. Br J Surg 29:407–414, 1942.

11. Stratford PW, Binkley J: A review of the McMurray test: Definition, interpretation, and clinical usefulness. J Orthop Sports Phys Ther 22:116–120, 1995.

12. Apley AG: The diagnosis of meniscus injuries. J Bone Joint Surg Br 29:78–84, 1947.

13. Hoppenfeld S: *Physical Examination of the Spine and Extremities.* Norwalk, CT, Appleton & Lange, 1976.

14. Hughston JC, Walsh WM, Puddu G: *Patellar Subluxation and Dislocation.* Philadelphia, WB Saunders, 1984.

15. Noble HB, Hajek MR, Porter M: Diagnosis and treatment of iliotibial band tightness in runners. Phys Sportsmed 10:67–74, 1982.

16. Ober FR: The role of the iliotibial band and fascia lata as a factor in the causation of low-back disabilities and sciatica. J Bone Joint Surg Am 18:105–110, 1936.

# Bibliography

Cherf J, Paulos LE: Bracing for patellar instability. Clin Sports Med 9:813–820, 1990.

Doucette SA, Goble EM: The effect of exercise on patellar tracking in lateral patellar compression syndrome. Am J Sports Med 20:434–440.

Ficat RP: *Disorders of the Patello-femoral Joint.* Baltimore, Williams & Wilkins, 1977.

Flynn TW, Soutas-Little RW: Patellofemoral joint compressive forces in forward and backward running. J Orthop Sports Phys Ther 21:277–281, 1985.

Hertling D, Kessler RM: *Management of Common Musculoskeletal Disorders: Physical Therapy Principles and Methods,* 2nd ed. Philadelphia, JB Lippincott, 1990.

Kisner C, Colby LA: *Therapeutic Exercise: Foundations and Techniques,* 2nd ed. Philadelphia, FA Davis, 1990.

McConnell J: The management of chondromalacia patellae: A long term solution. Aust J Physiother 32:215–223, 1986.

Noble HB, Hajek MR, Porter M: Diagnosis and treatment of iliotibial band tightness in runners. Phys Sportsmed 10:67–74, 1982.

Reider B, Sathy MR, Talkington J, et al: Treatment of isolated medial collateral ligament injuries in athletes with early functional rehabilitation: A five-year follow-up study. Am J Sports Med 22:470–477, 1993.

Thabit G, Micheli LJ: Patellofemoral pain in the pediatric patient. Orthop Clin North Am 23:567–585, 1992.

Tindel NL, Nisonson B: The plica syndrome. Orthop Clin North Am 23:613–618, 1992.

Zappala FG, Taffel CB, Scuderi GR: Rehabilitation of patellofemoral joint disorders. Orthop Clin North Am 23:555–566, 1992.

KNEE

9

# 10

# OOT AND ANKLE

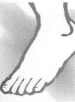

## Subjective Evaluation

▶ Pt Hx (region specific): Locking/ popping/ giving-way, type shoes/ wear pattern

▶ How does walking on various terrain affect swelling?

● For runners/joggers, how long has Pt been a jogger and what is jogging surface?

● Describe workout type/intensity/duration

# Objective Evaluation

I. Standing
  A. R/O spine pathology
  B. Observation
    1. Gait
    2. Posture (e.g., pes planus/cavus, calcaneal varus/valgus, genu varus/valgus/recurvatum, tibial torsion)
    3. Function
      a. Toe walking (S1–S2)
      b. Heel walking (L4–S1)
  C. GMMT
    1. Ankle PF (Single leg-heel raise[1]; test sidelying if status poor or worse)
II. Sitting
  A. Special tests (as applicable)
    1. Kleiger's test
III. Supine
  A. R/O knee, hip pathology
  B. Measure swelling/effusion
  C. AROM
    1. Ankle DF (10–15 deg)
    2. Ankle PF (45–55 deg)
    3. Ankle inv (30–40 deg)
    4. Ankle ev (15–25 deg)
  D. Special tests (as applicable)
    1. Ligament (ATFL): anterior drawer test
    2. Diastasis/syndesmotic sprain: squeeze test
    3. Stress fracture: metatarsal loading test
    4. Deep vein thrombophlebitis: Homans' sign
    5. Other: Morton's neuroma test
  E. Sensation
    1. Dermatomes (*see Appendix A*)
    2. Nerve fields

    F. Palpation
       1. Dorsal pedal and posterior tibial artery pulses
       2. Specific anatomic landmarks/ligaments
    G. Joint play: AP glide and long-axis distraction

IV. Sidelying
    A. GMMT
       1. Ankle inv/ev (test supine if status poor or worse)
    B. Special tests (as applicable)
       1. Ligament (CFL): talar tilt test
    C. Joint play
       1. Medial and lateral tilt tests

V. Prone
    A. Observation
       1. Posture (forefoot/rearfoot/varus/valgus)
    B. Special tests (as applicable)
       1. Ligament (ATFL): anterior drawer test
       2. Achilles tendon: Thompson's test

10 | FOOT AND ANKLE

## SPECIAL TESTS FOR THE FOOT AND ANKLE

| Test | Detects | Test Procedure | Positive Sign |
|------|---------|----------------|---------------|
| Single leg-heel raise[1] | Ankle PF strength | Pt standing on test limb with knee extended. Pt raises heel from floor through ROM of PF. | Test grades Normal and good: Pt completes four to five times with good form and no apparent fatigue Fair: Pt plantar flexes ankle sufficiently to clear heel from floor Poor and worse: Tested sidelying |
| Anterior drawer (ankle stability) test[2] | Compromised anterior talofibular lig | Pt prone with foot and ankle extending over edge of table and foot in 20 deg PF. Examiner stabilizes tibia and fibula and pushes calcaneus forward with other hand; this can also be performed with Pt sitting or supine and pulling calcaneus forward. | Increased anterior translation compared with uninvolved ankle. At same time, vacuum effect is seen in which skin on both sides of Achilles tendon is drawn inward (when sitting or supine, "dimples" may appear to form anteriorly because of vacuum effect). |
| Talar tilt (inv stress test)[3, 4] | Compromised calcaneofibular lig | Pt supine or sidelying. Pt's foot in neutral. Examiner tilts talus side to side in add and abd (inv and ev of foot). | Increase in talar tilt compared with uninvolved ankle, accompanied by lateral "dimpling" of skin around lat malleolus and soft end-feel |

| Kleiger's test[3] | Compromised deltoid lig (MCL) | Pt sitting with knee flexed over edge of table 90 deg. Examiner stabilizes leg with one hand and grasps foot and rotates it laterally (ER). | Med and lat pain, and examiner may feel talus displace from med malleolus |
|---|---|---|---|
| Squeeze test[4, 5] | Compromised interosseous lig, also known as syndesmotic ankle sprain | Pt sitting with leg over edge of table. Examiner places hands on Pt's leg approx 6 inches inferior to knee and compresses tibia and fibula with heels of both hands, as if to bring them together, and then releases | Exquisite pain reproduced during test in vicinity of distal syndesmosis or ankle joint |
| ER stress test[6] | Compromised interosseous lig, also known as syndesmotic ankle sprain | Pt sitting with leg over edge of table and knee flexed 90 deg and ankle in neutral position. Examiner applies ER stress to involved foot and ankle. | Exquisite pain reproduced over anterior or posterior tibiofibular lig and over interosseous membrane |
| Homans' sign[3] | Deep vein thrombophlebitis | Examiner palpates deep between heads of Pt's gastrocnemius or forcibly dorsiflexes Pt's ankle when knee is fully extended | Exquisite pain in calf |

*Continued*

# SPECIAL TESTS FOR THE FOOT AND ANKLE *Continued*

| Test | Detects | Test Procedure | Positive Sign |
|------|---------|----------------|---------------|
| Thompson's test[7] | Ruptured Achilles tendon | Pt gets in quadruped position (on all fours) on table. Examiner squeezes calf (med and lat sides of gastrocnemius). | Absence of ankle PF (present but significantly reduced PF may represent partial tear) |
| Vibration test | Stress Fx | Examiner places tuning fork on suspected stress Fx site. Ultrasound (100%) over suspected stress Fx may also be used for similar effect. | Exquisite pain at suspected stress Fx site |
| Metatarsal loading test | Stress Fx in metatarsal | Examiner grasps metatarsal head with fingers and pushes it toward calcaneus (axial loading). | Reproduction of Pt's Sx |
| Test for Morton's neuroma[8] | Morton's neuroma | Examiner grasps two metatarsal heads, between which is the suspected neuroma. Examiner moves metatarsal heads back and forth while compressing them together. | Reproduction of Pt's Sx (e.g., exquisite pain, burning, shooting, tingling) |

| Special Condition | Hx/Symptoms | Signs/Objective Findings | Treatment Options |
|---|---|---|---|
| Achilles tendinitis, acute | Painful Achilles tendon, crepitus<br>Pt reports increased Sx with running, jumping, stair climbing<br>Rest decreases Sx | Achilles tendon tender to palpation<br>Heel raises and forced ankle DF reproduces Sx | Relative rest, ice, heel lift, NSAIDs, phonophoresis/iontophoresis<br>*Subacute:* gentle calf stretching, transverse friction massage (TFM); may consider eccentric training program after Sx subside (SAID)<br>Correct biomechanical problems that may be contributing |
| Achilles tendinitis, chronic | Chronic achilles tendon pain (Pt may have continued to exercise through pain for months) | Nodules in achilles tendon<br>May have partial rupture<br>Remember to perform Thompson's test for both acute and chronic conditions | Heel lift, TFM<br>May require 4–6 mo of decreased activity<br>Calf stretching<br>Strengthening anterior muscle group<br>May consider eccentric training program (SAID)<br>Correct biomechanical problems that may be contributing<br>May require surgery if no improvement |

*Continued* ▶

| Special Condition | Hx/Symptoms | Signs/Objective Findings | Treatment Options |
|---|---|---|---|
| Achilles tendon rupture | H/O rapid eccentric loading (e.g., jumping, sprinting, stair climbing)<br>Severe pain in achilles tendon<br>Pt may report hearing a "pop" or feeling as though struck from behind at time of injury | Positive Thompson's test<br>Observable gap may be present beneath skin between ends of ruptured tendon in midsubstance rupture<br>Exquisite tenderness at rupture site whether it is midsubstance or at insertion into calcaneus<br>Pt unable to perform a toe raise on involved LE | Refer Pt to orthopedic surgeon<br>Pt may be treated operatively or nonoperatively<br>*Nonoperative Rx:* involves casting in PF (6–10 wk) initially. After cast removed, Rx aimed at restoring AROM. Strengthening is then also progressed carefully from isometrics through isotonics and isokinetics. Eccentric loading/strengthening should also be part of later stages of rehabilitation. Some authorities do not recommend this option for an active, athletic patient[9]<br>*Possible rehabilitation approach after operative Rx:*<br>  Week 1: ice, NWB, AROM out of splint<br>  Week 2: ice, NWB, AROM out of splint, isometric inv/ev, gather towel with toes, mobilize scar<br>  Week 3: begin PWB in cam-walker or cast with walking boot; if no cast, AROM, |

| Plantar fasciitis | Often coexists with calcaneal spurs<br>Pain in AM with first few steps | Tender over plantar foot and/or plantar calcaneus | gentle calf/Achilles stretch with towel, isometric PF/DF/inv/ev, begin light isotonic PF/DF/inv/ev with tubing (10 repetitions)<br>Week 4–6: progress PWB up to FWB by week 6, AROM, progress calf/achilles stretching (may begin standing stretch), progress isotonic strengthening, proprioception<br>Week 6–12: FWB in footwear with high heel such as boots, progress stretching, continue isotonics and add toe raises with both LEs<br>Week 12 +: progress all exercises and prudently progress walk to jog; pool exercises<br>Use modalities as needed to assist rehab<br>Decrease activity, NSAIDs, phonophoresis/iontophoresis<br>Orthoses/low-dye taping<br>Plantar fascia, gastrocnemius, and soleus muscle stretch<br>Pt education to wear supportive shoes at all times and avoid walking barefoot or in sandals<br>Night splints for recalcitrant cases |

*Continued*

131

**TREATMENT OPTIONS FOR THE FOOT AND ANKLE** *Continued*

| Special Condition | Hx/Symptoms | Signs/Objective Findings | Treatment Options |
|---|---|---|---|
| Stress Fx | Vague insidious onset of Sx<br>Localized tenderness over bone<br>Pain subsides with rest<br>An overuse injury | Common areas are metatarsals, tibia, calcaneus<br>Tender directly over bone<br>Positive metatarsal loading or vibration tests | Rest<br>Prescribe appropriate ambulatory status based on Pt's Sx during weight bearing<br>NWB exercise initially, progressing to weight-bearing exercise as Sx resolve<br>Ensure Pt obtaining proper/sufficient nutrition |
| Compartment syndrome, acute (medical emergency) | Disproportionate pain with passive stretch<br>Paresthesia<br>Muscle weakness<br>Progresses rapidly (in 8–12 hr can cause permanent damage) | Associated with severe trauma (Fx), burns, and excessive overuse | Elevate to horizontal<br>Monitor closely<br>Notify physician/orthopedic surgeon immediately |
| Compartment syndrome, chronic/exercise induced | Similar to acute but less intense pain<br>No rapid progress<br>Sx subside with rest | Associated with activity/exercise | Increase flexibility<br>Increase muscle endurance<br>Correct mechanical fault<br>Surgical release if continually problematic |

| | | | |
|---|---|---|---|
| Ankle sprain, grade I and II* | H/O trauma (inv or ev force)<br>Mild to moderate pain and disability | Swelling<br>Tenderness over LCL (ATFL, CFL, PTFL) in inv injury or MCL/deltoid lig (TNL, ATTL, TCL, PTTL) in ev injury<br>May or may not have positive anterior drawer test or talar tilt test with laxity present, but definite firm end-feel<br>Assess for presence of syndesmosis sprain and R/O osteochondral Fx of talar dome | *Acute:* reduce swelling (ice, elevate, compression tape/wrap, NSAIDs), crutches to reduce weight bearing<br>*Subacute:* AROM (alphabet, pumping, inv, ev), isometric strengthening (DF, PF, inv, ev), wean from crutches<br>*Chronic:* Isotonic strengthening (DF, PF, inv, ev), calf stretch, balance/proprioceptive training, agility/return to sport activity |
| Ankle sprain, grade III* | H/O trauma (inv or ev force)<br>Severe pain and disability | Swelling<br>Tenderness over lig comprising LCL (inv) or MCL/deltoid lig (ev)<br>Positive anterior drawer test and talar tilt test both with soft/empty end-feel with LCL sprain<br>Positive Kleiger's test with MCL sprain<br>Assess for presence of syndesmosis sprain and R/O osteochondral Fx of talar dome | *Acute:* reduce swelling (ice, elevate, compression tape/wrap, NSAIDs), crutches to reduce weight bearing, ankle stirrup brace<br>*Subacute:* AROM (alphabet, pumping, inv, ev), isometric strengthening (DF, PF, inv, ev), wean from crutches<br>*Chronic:* isotonic strengthening (DF, PF, inv, ev), calf stretch, balance/proprioceptive training, lace-up ankle brace for support in return to sport activities, agility/return to sport activity<br>If aggressive nonoperative Fx fails to restore stability, reconstructive surgery may be required |

*Continued*

133

**TREATMENT OPTIONS FOR THE FOOT AND ANKLE** *Continued*

| Special Condition | Hx/Symptoms | Signs/Objective Findings | Treatment Options |
|---|---|---|---|
| Syndesmosis sprain | MOI described as ER force or hyperdorsiflexion force to foot/ankle<br>Swelling usually less prominent in these injuries than in lat ankle sprains | Tenderness over anterior tibiofibular lig, proximal to anterior talofibular lig<br>Tenderness over syndesmosis or posterior tibiofibular lig | Similar to ankle sprain rehabilitation described earlier. Remember that these injuries take significantly more time to heal<br><br>*Acute:* reduce swelling (ice, elevate, compression tape/wrap, NSAIDs), crutches to reduce weight bearing, ankle stirrup brace<br><br>*Subacute:* AROM (alphabet, pumping, inv, ev), isometric strengthening (DF, PF, inv, ev), wean from crutches<br><br>*Chronic:* isotonic strengthening (DF, PF, inv, ev), calf stretch, balance/proprioceptive training, lace-up ankle brace for support in return to sport activities, agility/return to sport activity |
| Morton's neuroma | Burning/shooting pain between metatarsals/metatarsal heads<br>Pain radiates from metatarsal heads into toes | Positive Morton's neuroma test | Support transverse arch<br>Have Pt wear a wider shoe<br>May require referral to podiatrist for local steroid injection or surgical excision of neuroma |

*See Appendix E for standard nomenclature of athletic injuries.

# References

1. Daniels L, Worthingham C: *Muscle Testing: Techniques of Manual Examination*, 5th ed. Philadelphia, WB Saunders, 1986.

2. Gungor T: A test for ankle instability: A brief report. J Bone Joint Surg Br 70:487, 1988.

3. Magee DJ: *Orthopedic Physical Assessment*, 3rd ed. Philadelphia, WB Saunders, 1997.

4. Trevino SG, Davis P, Hecht PJ: Management of acute and chronic lateral ligament injuries of the ankle. Orthop Clin North Am 25:1–16, 1994.

5. Swain RA, Holt WS: Ankle injuries: Tips from sports medicine physicians. Postgrad Med 93:91–100, 1993.

6. Boytim MJ, Fischer DA, Neumann L: Syndesmotic ankle sprains. Am J Sports Med 19:294–298, 1991.

7. Kelikian H, Kelikian AS: *Disorders of the Ankle*. Philadelphia, WB Saunders, 1985.

8. Calliet R: *Foot and Ankle Pain*, 2nd ed. Philadelphia, FA Davis, 1983.

9. Cetti R, Christensen S, Ejsted R, et al: Operative versus nonoperative treatment of Achilles tendon rupture. Am J Sports Med 21:791–799, 1993.

# Bibliography

Boytim MJ, Fischer DA, Neumann L: Syndesmotic ankle sprains. Am J Sports Med 19:294–298.

Calliet R: *Foot and Ankle Pain*, 2nd ed. Philadelphia, FA Davis, 1983.

Clement DB, Taunton JE, Smart GW: Achilles tendinitis and peritendinitis: Etiology and treatment. Am J Sports Med 12:179–184, 1984.

Cox JS: Surgical and nonsurgical treatment of acute ankle sprains. Clin Orthop 198:118–126, 1985.

Curwin S, Stanish WD: *Tendinitis: Its Etiology and Treatment*. Lexington, MA, DC Heath, 1984.

Galloway MT, Jokl P, Dayton OW: Achilles tendon overuse injuries. Clin Sports Med 11:771–780, 1992.

Hertling D, Kessler RM: *Management of Common Musculoskeletal Disorders: Physical Therapy Principles and Methods*, 2nd ed. Philadelphia, JB Lippincott, 1990.

Mascaro TB, Swanson LE: Rehabilitation of the foot and ankle. Orthop Clin North Am 25:147–160, 1994.

Schepsis AA, Leach RE, Goryca J: Plantar fasciitis: Etiology, treatment, surgical results, and review of the literature. Clin Orthop 266:185–196, 1991.

Seto JL, Brewster CE: Treatment approaches following foot and ankle injury. Clin Sports Med 13:695–718, 1994.

Soma CA, Mandelbaum BR: Repair of acute Achilles tendon ruptures. Orthop Clin North Am 26:239–247, 1995.

Swain RA, Holt WS: Ankle injuries: Tips from sports medicine physicians. Postgrad Med 93:91–100, 1993.

Trevino SG, Davis P, Hecht PJ: Management of acute and chronic lateral ligament injuries of the ankle. Orthop Clin North Am 25:1–16, 1994.

Wapner KL, Sharkey PF: The use of night splints for treatment of recalcitrant plantar fasciitis. Foot Ankle 12:135–137, 1991.

# 11

# RESPIRATORY EVALUATION

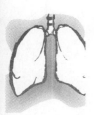

## Subjective Evaluation

▶ Pt Hx (respiratory specific): age, sex, diagnosis, vital signs, swallowing, nutritional status, chest radiographs, PFT tests, laboratory reports on sputum, cough

▶ Smoking Hx, other environmental factors/exposures

▶ Family/support system

# Objective Evaluation

I. Observation
   A. Posture
   B. Use of accessory muscles
   C. Furrowed brow
   D. Flaring nares
   E. Pursed-lip breathing
   F. Increased work to breathe
   G. Respiratory rate and depth
   H. Cyanosis/clubbing of nails
   I. Pt's color (e.g., pallor, red, blue)
   J. Supplemental devices (e.g., oxygen, ventilator)
   K. Oxygen saturation (no exercise if <90%)
II. Chest assessment
   A. Chest shape/size
   B. Tone
   C. Upright posturing
III. Breathing pattern
   A. Brain stem involvement
   B. Diaphragmatic
   C. Paradoxic
   D. Diaphragm only
   E. Upper accessory muscles only
   F. Asymmetric
   G. Shallow
   H. Irregular
   I. Work of breathing
IV. Phonation
   A. Length
   B. Voice intensity/quality
   C. Listen with the stethoscope for abnormal vocal resonance

V. Cough
   A. Inspiration
   B. Force buildup
   C. Expulsion
   D. Production
VI. Manual assessment
   A. Vital signs
   B. Auscultation (e.g., abnormal breath sounds, rales, wheezing, pleural friction rub)
   C. PFTs (VC, $V_t$, $FEV_1$, FRC)
   D. Chest wall expansion measurement (i.e., level of axilla, fourth intercostal space, nipple line, and 10th rib)
VII. Palpation
   A. Check
      1. Chest/thoracic and abdominal asymmetries
      2. Abnormal contours
      3. Lumps
      4. Masses
      5. Soft tissue swelling
      6. Efficacy of muscle contraction
   B. Percussion (i.e., placing finger over intercostal spaces at symmetric lung segments from apex to base and tapping with opposite finger at each site): Is the sound resonant, dull, or flat?
   C. Pitting edema in the LEs
VIII. Function
   A. Monitor response when Pt is allowed activity (e.g., walking, wheel chair propulsion, ADLs)

RESPIRATORY EVALUATION 11

## Bibliography

Cohen M, Michel TH: *Cardiopulmonary Symptoms in Physical Therapy Practice*. New York, Churchill Livingstone, 1988.

Hobson L, Hammon WE: Chest assessment. In Frownfelter DL (ed): *Chest Physical Therapy and Pulmonary Rehabilitation: An Interdisciplinary Approach*, 2nd ed. Chicago, Year Book Medical Publishers, 1987.

Scanlan CL: Chest physical therapy. In Scanlan CL, Spearman CB, Sheldon RL (eds): *Egan's Fundamentals of Respiratory Care*, 5th ed. St. Louis, CV Mosby, 1990.

Wilkins RL: Physical assessment of the patient. In Scanlan CL, Spearman CB, Sheldon RL (eds): *Egan's Fundamentals of Respiratory Care*, 5th ed. St. Louis, CV Mosby, 1990.

Youtsey JW: Basic pulmonary function measurements. In Scanlan CL, Spearman CB, Sheldon RL (eds): *Egan's Fundamentals of Respiratory Care*, 5th ed. St. Louis, CV Mosby, 1990.

Zadai CC: Comprehensive physical therapy evaluation: Identifying potential pulmonary limitations. In Zadai CC (ed): *Pulmonary Management in Physical Therapy*. New York, Churchill Livingstone, 1992.

**12**

# INPATIENT PHYSICAL THERAPY
# CARDIAC EVALUATION

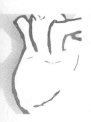

## Subjective Evaluation

▶ Pt Hx (cardiac specific): age, sex, diagnosis

▶ Are any Sx present today (chest/neck/left shoulder/jaw pain; syncope or dizziness)?

▶ Does Pt feel "palpitation" of the heart (i.e., "pounding, stopping, jumping, or racing" in the chest), fever, or chills?

▶ Laboratory and ECG results

▶ Has Pt had surgical intervention?

▶ Nutritional status, smoking Hx, PMHx, PSHx, Meds

▶ Other significant cardiac risk factors

# Objective Evaluation

I. Observation
   A. General appearance: Does Pt look ill?
   B. Edema in the extremities
   C. Posture (i.e., sternal or spinal deformities that may affect the heart)
   D. Cyanosis/clubbing of nails
   E. Supplemental devices (e.g., oxygen, ventilator)
   F. Congenital abnormalities

II. Vital signs
   A. Blood pressure: record blood pressure and pulse while Pt is sitting or reclining, standing before exercising, and during and after exercises/ambulation (if Pt is stable and has been cleared by physician to begin cardiac rehabilitation)
   B. Pulse (beats per minute and regularity)
   C. Auscultation

III. Breathing pattern
   A. Dyspnea
   B. Wheezing
   C. Orthopnea
   D. Cheyne-Stokes breathing
   E. Overuse of accessory muscles
   F. Increased work of breathing

IV. Phonation
   A. Length
   B. Voice intensity/quality
   C. Listen with the stethoscope for abnormal vocal resonance

V. Cough
   A. Inspiration
   B. Force buildup

C. Expulsion

D. Production (color of sputum)

VI. Function

   A. Bed mobility

   B. Transfers

   C. Ambulation

## Bibliography

Goldberger E: *Essentials of Clinical Cardiology.* Philadelphia, JB Lippincott, 1990.

Hurst JW, Crawley IS, Morris DC, Dorney ER: The history: Symptoms and past events related to cardiovascular disease. In Hurst JW, Schlant RC, Rackley CE, Sonnenblick EH, Wenger NK (eds): *The Heart: Arteries and Veins*, 7th ed, vol 1. New York, McGraw-Hill, 1990:122–134.

Silverman ME: Inspection of the patient. In Hurst JW, Schlant RC, Rackley CE, Sonnenblick EH, Wenger NK (eds): *The Heart: Arteries and Veins*, 7th ed, vol 1. New York, McGraw-Hill, 1990:135–147.

Willerson JT: Physical examination of the patient with heart disease. In Sanford JP, Willerson JT, Sanders CA (eds): *The Science and Practice of Clinical Medicine: Clinical Cardiology*, vol 3. New York, Grune & Stratton, 1977:94–111.

CARDIAC EVALUATION

12

# OWER EXTREMITY AMPUTATION EVALUATION

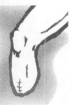

## Subjective Evaluation

▶ Pt Hx (amputation specific): age, sex, date and type of amputation, present MHx

▶ Motivation, communication abilities, family support

Home specifics (e.g., stairs, type of carpet, bathroom layout)

Lifestyle

Pt's goals for therapy

# Objective Evaluation

I. Observation

   A. Vital signs

   B. Skin: wound healing, perspiration, check for trophic changes

   C. Shape: conical, cylindrical, bulbous, edematous, dog ears

   D. Measurements: girth, length

   E. Circulation: pulses, coloration

   F. Motor function: strength, tone of all extremities

   G. Sensation

      1. Light touch, hot/cold, sharp, proprioception, phantom sensation

      2. Educate Pt about importance of desensitization of residual limb to tapping or rubbing

   H. Pain

      1. Bone, vascular, nerve, wound, phantom pain

      2. Frequency, intensity, duration, description

   I. ROM for all joints: note any contractures

      1. Common AKA contractures: hip flex, ER, abd

      2. Common BKA contractures: hip flex, ER, abd, knee flex

   J. Function

      1. Bed mobility

      2. Balance (sitting, standing)

      3. Transfers (sit-to-stand and bed-to-wheelchair, each with and without the prosthesis)

      4. Gait (amount of weight bearing, assistive devices, tolerance, stairs)

   K. ADLs

1. Bath, dressing, toilet, bandaging of residual limb independently
2. Donning/doffing of the prosthesis independently

## Bibliography

Karacoloff LA, Hammersley CS, Schneider FJ: *Lower Extremity Amputation: A Guide to Functional Outcomes in Physical Therapy Management*. Gaithersburg, MD, Aspen, 1992.
Skinner HB, Effeney DJ: Gait analysis in amputees. Am J Phys Med 64:82–89, 1985.

# 14

# NEUROLOGIC EVALUATION

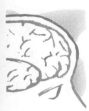

## Subjective Evaluation

▶ Pt Hx (neurologic specific): onset of present condition, diagnosis, test results, precautions

▶ Home environment (e.g., barriers), family support

▶ Recovery to date, Pt's goals

# Objective Evaluation

I. Observations
   A. Catheter
   B. Oxygen
   C. Intravenous lines
   D. Ventilator or other assistive devices
II. Mental status
   A. State of consciousness (e.g., alert, lethargic, obtunded, stupor, coma)
   B. Score on standardized cognitive function scale
   C. Orientation (person/place/time) x 1, 2, 3
   D. Memory (short and long term)
   E. Attention
   F. Calculation
   G. Abstract thinking
III. Communication
   A. Aphasia: global or Wernicke's (receptive), Broca's (expressive)
   B. Observe Pt's ability to name objects, write, read aloud, and follow directions
   C. Establish method of communicating with Pt
IV. Cranial nerves (see Special Tests table)
V. Reflexes
   A. MSRs
   B. Pathologic
      1. Clonus
      2. Babinski's sign or reflex
      3. Hoffmann's sign
      4. Other superficial or postural reflexes
VI. Sensation
   A. Light touch
   B. Pain
   C. Proprioception
   D. Combined sensations

1. Stereognosis
2. Tactile localization
3. Two-point discrimination
4. Bilateral, simultaneous stimulation (e.g., vibration)

VII. Skin

A. Check to ensure no decubiti forming

VIII. Perception

A. Spatial neglect
B. Apraxia
C. Agnosia

IX. Musculoskeletal

A. Involuntary movement (e.g., tremor, chorea, athetosis)
B. Muscle tone (e.g., spasticity, rigidity, flaccidity)
C. PROM and AROM

X. Respiratory

A. Airway protection, mechanics, cough

XI. Coordination

A. Finger-to-nose test
B. Pronation/supination (rapid alternating movements)
C. Alternate nose-to-finger test

XII. Balance

A. Static and dynamic
B. Sitting and standing (e.g., Romberg's test, functional reach, perturbation testing)

XIII. ADLs*

A. Bed mobility
B. Sit-to-stand movement
C. Transfers
D. Gait

14 | NEUROLOGIC EVALUATION

---

* Compile a problem list, with short- and long-term goals, and a treatment plan. Educate the family about positioning, bed mobility, transfers, and safety.

## SPECIAL TESTS FOR NEUROLOGIC EVALUATION

| Test | Detects | Test Procedure | Positive Sign |
|------|---------|----------------|---------------|
| Cranial nerve function[1] | Which areas of central nervous system may be involved by assessing functions of cranial nerves | I: olfactory (sense of smell)<br>II: optic (visual field)<br>III, IV, VI: pupillary reaction to light, extraocular muscle function (look up, down, and side to side)<br>V: trigeminal (bilateral simultaneous stimulation with pin or light touch to face)<br>VII: facial (smile, frown, wrinkle brow)<br>VIII: auditory and vestibular (hearing, vertigo)<br>IX, X: glossopharyngeal and vagus (gag reflex)<br>XI: accessory (trapezius/shoulder shrug, SCM)<br>XII: hypoglossal (tongue protrusion) | Loss or asymmetry of any of these functions/reflexes |
| Babinski's reflex/sign[2] | Upper motor neuron lesion | Pt supine. Examiner runs pointed object along plantar aspect of Pt's foot and across metatarsal heads lat to med | Pt involuntarily extends big toe and abducts (splays) other toes |
| Hoffmann's sign[2] (pathologic reflex for UE, similar to Babinski's sign for LE) | Upper motor neuron lesion/ corticospinal tract lesion of spinal cord | Examiner grasps and stabilizes Pt's hand and "flicks" distal phalanx of Pt's middle finger in direction of ext, causing quick stretch of finger flexors | Induced flex of thumb and other fingers |

| | | | |
|---|---|---|---|
| Clonus[2] | Upper motor neuron lesion | Pt sitting with knees flexed and hanging over edge of exam table. Examiner places a quick stretch on gastrocnemius muscle by abruptly moving Pt's foot upward (into DF). | Rapid oscillations of contraction and relaxation occur in response to this quick stretch, causing reverberating DF/PF motion of ankle. There may be several beats or, in some cases, clonus does not cease until stretch is released when examiner passively plantar flexes Pt's ankle |
| Pupillary light reflex[1] | Lesion of cranial nerve II or III | Examiner shines light into one eye of Pt | Lesion of cranial nerve III on test side: pupil of eye on test side into which light is shined fails to constrict and opposite pupil does constrict when light is shined into opposite side, only that pupil constricts<br>Lesion of cranial nerve II on test side: neither pupil constricts when light is shined into eye on test side, but both pupils constrict when light is shined into opposite eye |
| Gag reflex[1] | Lesion of cranial nerve IX or X | Examiner uses tongue depressor to touch soft palate or pharynx | Asymmetry in retraction of soft palate during gag. Palate retracts to normal side (away from side of central nervous system lesion). |

*Continued* ▶

153

## SPECIAL TESTS FOR NEUROLOGIC EVALUATION Continued

| Test | Detects | Test Procedure | Positive Sign |
|------|---------|----------------|---------------|
| Romberg's test[3] | Vestibular dysfunction/balance deficit | Pt standing with feet together and eyes closed. Examiner observes and notes postural reaction. | Excessive postural sway, tendency to fall to one side, abd of arms more to one side than other, and associated movements of mouth and hands |
| Coordination tests[4] | Cerebellar dysfunction | *Finger-to-nose:* Pt's shoulder abducted 90 deg with elbow extended. Pt then asked to touch tip of index finger to tip of nose. | Difficulty or inability to perform on one side compared with opposite side |
| | | *Alternate nose-to-finger:* Pt alternately touches tip of nose and tip of examiner's finger using index finger. Examiner may change positions of finger in front of Pt to assess Pt's ability to change distance, direction, and force of movement. | Difficulty or inability to perform on one side compared with opposite side |
| | | *Pronation/supination:* have Pt hold arms into sides with elbows flexed 90 deg. Then have Pt alternately pronate/supinate forearms/hands, gradually increasing speed. | Inability to coordinate hands so they perform pronation/supination alternately, and/or inability to perform test rapidly |

## References

1. Goldberg SG: *The 4-minute Neurologic Exam*. Miami, FL, MedMaster, 1992.

2. Dodd J, Kelly JP: Trigeminal system. In Kandel ER, Schwartz JH, Jessell TM (eds): *Principles of Neural Science*, 3rd ed. New York, Elsevier Science Publishing, 1991.

3. Cermak SA, Henderson A: Learning disabilities. In Umphred DA (ed): *Neurological Rehabilitation*, 2nd ed. St. Louis, CV Mosby, 1990.

4. Schmitz TJ: Coordination assessment. In O'Sullivan SB, Schmitz TJ (eds): *Physical Rehabilitation: Assessment and Treatment*, 2nd ed. Philadelphia, FA Davis, 1988.

## Bibliography

Goldberg SG: *The 4-minute Neurologic Exam*. Miami, FL, MedMaster, 1992.

O'Sullivan SB, Schmitz TJ: *Physical Rehabilitation: Assessment and Treatment*, 2nd ed. Philadelphia, FA Davis, 1988.

Umphred DA (ed): *Neurological Rehabilitation*, 2nd ed. St. Louis, CV Mosby, 1990.

# 15

# INPATIENT ORTHOPEDIC EVALUATION

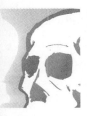

## Subjective Evaluation

- Pt Hx (inpatient orthopedic specific)
- Surgery/diagnosis: procedure and date, postsurgical complications, EBL, expected discharge date
- Presurgical functional level
- Home environment (e.g., carpet, stairs) and living arrangements, if applicable
- Meds, radiograph/CT/MRI

# Objective Evaluation

I. Vital signs, temperature, oxygen saturation
II. Mental status
III. Gait, if applicable
IV. AROM and PROM, if applicable
V. Strength of upper and lower extremity, as applies
VI. Sensation
   A. Light touch
   B. Sharp/dull
   C. Two-point discrimination
VII. Reflexes
   A. MSRs
   B. Pathologic
      1. Babinski's reflex present/not present
      2. Clonus present/not present and number of beats
VIII. Vascular
   A. Pulses
      1. Radial
      2. DP
      3. PT
      4. Capillary refill in finger/toenail beds
      5. Extremity temperature
IX. Balance, if applicable
   A. Romberg's test
   B. Sitting and standing with perturbation
   C. Single-leg stance
   D. Dynamic balance during gait
X. Coordination, if applicable
   A. Finger-nose-finger test
   B. Heel-to-shin test
   C. Rapid alternating movements

XI. Special tests, if applicable

XII. Palpation, if applicable

XIII. Functional assessment

   A. Bed mobility
   B. Transfers
   C. Ambulation

# APPENDIX A

## Dermatomes

The dermatomes follow a highly regular pattern on the body. S, sacral; L, lumbar; T, thoracic; C, cervical. In actuality, the boundaries of the dermatomes are less distinct than shown here because of overlapping innervation.

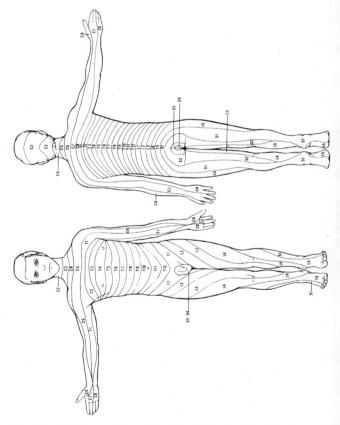

Reproduced with permission from Kandel ER: *Principles of Neural Science*, 3rd ed. New York, Elsevier Publishers, 1991.

# APPENDIX B

## Sclerotomes

The sclerotomes are areas of bone or fascia that are supplied by individual nerve roots.

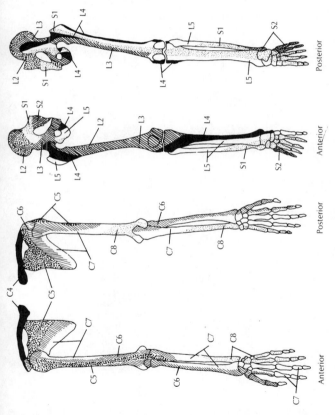

B ▮ SCLEROTOMES

# APPENDIX C

## Auscultation

The patient is asked to breathe through his mouth, slowly and easily, deeper than normal. A right-to-left sequence is used, always comparing one side with the other *(A, B)*. New examiners should listen to several "normal" chests to get a baseline for what is abnormal *(C, D)*.

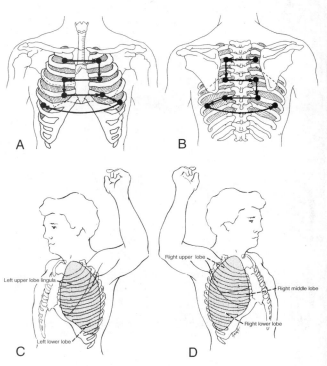

*A,* Path of auscultation on the anterior chest. *B,* Path of auscultation on the posterior chest. *C* and *D,* Relationship of the lung to surface anatomy. The examiner must consider the lung areas being auscultated. (From Frownfelter DL (ed): *Chest Physical Therapy and Pulmonary Rehabilitation,* 2nd ed. St. Louis, Mosby–Year Book, 1978.)

# APPENDIX D

Normal Range of Motion*

| | Wiechec and Krusen[1] | Dorinson and Wagner[2] | JAMA[3] | Daniels and Worthingham[4] | Esch and Lepley[5] | Gerhardt and Russe[6] | Boone and Azen[7,‡] | AAOS[8] | CMA[9] | Clarke[10] |
|---|---|---|---|---|---|---|---|---|---|---|
| **Shoulder†** | | | | | | | | | | |
| Flexion | 180 | 180 | 150 | 90[a] | 170 | 170 | 167 | 180 | 170 | 130 |
| Extension | 45 | 45 | 40 | 50 | 60 | 50 | 62 | 60 | 30 | 80 |
| Abduction | 180 | 180 | 150 | 90[a] | 170 | 170 | 184 | 180 | 170 | 180 |
| Internal rotation | 90 | 90 | 40[b] | 90 | 80 | 80 | 69 | 70 | 60[b] | 90[b] |
| External rotation | 90 | 90 | 90[b] | 90 | 90 | 90 | 104 | 90 | 80[b] | 40[b] |
| Horizontal abduction | | | | | | 30 | 45 | | | |
| Horizontal adduction | | | | | | 135 | 140 | 135 | | |
| **Elbow** | | | | | | | | | | |
| Flexion | 135 | 145 | 150 | 160 | 150 | 150 | 143 | 150 | 135 | 150 |
| Pronation | 90 | 80 | 80 | 90 | 90 | 80 | 76 | 80 | 75 | 50 |
| Supination | 90 | 70 | 80 | 90 | 90 | 90 | 82 | 80 | 85 | 90 |
| **Wrist** | | | | | | | | | | |
| Flexion | 60 | 80 | 70 | 90 | 90 | 60 | 76 | 80 | 70 | 80 |
| Extension | 55 | 55 | 60 | 90 | 70 | 50 | 75 | 70 | 65 | 70 |
| Radial deviation | 35 | 20 | 20 | 25 | 20 | 20 | 22 | 20 | 20 | 15 |
| Ulnar deviation | 75 | 40 | 30 | 65 | 30 | 30 | 36 | 30 | 40 | 30 |

| | | | | | | | | | | |
|---|---|---|---|---|---|---|---|---|---|---|
| **Hip** | | | | | | | | | | |
| Flexion | 120 | 125 | 100 | 125 | 130 | 125 | 122 | 120 | 110 | 120 |
| Extension | 45 | 50 | 30 | 15 | 45 | 15 | 10 | 30 | 30 | 20 |
| Abduction | 45 | 45 | 40 | 45 | 45 | 45 | 46 | 45 | 50 | 55 |
| Adduction | | 20 | 20 | 0 | 15 | 15 | 27 | 30 | 30 | 45 |
| Internal rotation | | 30 | 40 | 45 | 33 | 45 | 47 | 45 | 35 | 20 |
| External rotation | | 50 | 50 | 45 | 36 | 45 | 47 | 45 | 50 | 45 |
| **Knee** | | | | | | | | | | |
| Flexion | 135 | 140 | 120 | 130 | 135 | 130 | 143 | 135 | 135 | 145 |
| **Ankle** | | | | | | | | | | |
| Plantar flexion | 55 | 45 | 40 | 45 | 65 | 45 | 56 | 50 | 50 | 50 |
| Dorsiflexion | 30 | 20 | 20 | | 10 | 20 | 13 | 20 | 15 | 15 |
| Inversion | | 50 | 30 | | 30 | 40 | 37 | 35 | 35 | |
| Eversion | | 20 | 20 | | 15 | 20 | 26 | 15 | 20 | |

*These "normal" values (in degrees) are associated with manual muscle testing, and the authors list only the part of the movement attributable to the deltoid muscle. As demonstrated by this table, published normal range of motion values vary. Normal ranges of motion were derived primarily from Daniels L, Worthingham C. *Muscle Testing: Techniques of Manual Examination*, 5th ed. Philadelphia: W.B. Saunders Co., 1986.

†Tested with the shoulder in 0 degrees of abduction.

‡This is the only article in which the methodology for obtaining normal values was reported. The values presented represent the means of measurements taken on 109 men ranging in age from 18 months to 54 years.

Reproduced with permission from Rothstein JM (ed). *Measurement in Physical Therapy*. New York, Churchill Livingstone, 1985.

## References

1. Wiechec FJ, Krusen FH: A new method of joint measurement and a review of the literature. Am J Surg 43:659, 1939.

2. Dorinson SM, Wagner ML: An exact technic for clinically measuring and recording joint motion. Arch Phys Med 29:468, 1948.

3. A guide to the evaluation of permanent impairment of the extremities and back. JAMA Special ed:1, 1958.

4. Daniels L, Worthingham C: *Muscle testing. Techniques of Manual Examination*, 5th ed. Philadelphia, WB Saunders, 1986.

5. Esch D, Lepley M: *Evaluation of Joint Motion: Methods of Measurement and Recording*. Minneapolis, University of Minnesota Press, 1974.

6. Gerhardt JJ, Russe OA: *International SFTR Method of Measuring and Recording Joint Motion*. Bern, Huber, 1975.

7. Boone DC, Azen SP: Normal range of motion of joints in male subjects. J Bone Joint Surg Am 61a:756–759, 1979.

8. American Academy of Orthopaedic Surgeons: *Joint Motion: Method of Measuring and Recording*. Chicago, American Academy of Orthopaedic Surgeons, 1965.

9. Commission of California Medical Association and The Industrial Accident Commission of the State of California: *Evaluation of Industrial Disability*. New York, Oxford University Press, 1960.

10. Clarke WA: A system of joint measurement. J Orthop Surg 2:687, 1920.

# APPENDIX E

## Ligament Laxity Grading Scale

**Grade I/First-Degree/Mild Sprain.** Tear of a minimum number of fibers of the ligament and local tenderness but no instability. Joint surfaces separate 5 mm or less during stress testing.

**Grade II/Second-Degree/Moderate Sprain.** Tear of more fibers and more generalized tenderness but no gross instability. Joint surfaces separate 5–10 mm during stress testing.

**Grade III/Third-Degree/Severe Sprain.** Complete rupture of the ligament with gross instability. Joint surfaces separate 10 mm or more.

Data from Committee on the Medical Aspects of Sports of the American Medical Association: Standard Nomenclature of Athletic Injuries. Chicago, American Medical Association, 1976.

# APPENDIX F

## Capsular Pattern and Closed Pack Positions for Selected Joints

| Joints | Capsular Pattern | Closed Pack Position |
|---|---|---|
| Cervical spine | lat flex and ER | ext (facet joints) |
| Shoulder | ER, abd, IR | |
| Elbow | flex, ext | |
| Wrist | equal all motions | full ext |
| Carpometacarpal | abd, ext | full opposition |
| MCP | flex, ext | 1st MCP, full opposition |
| | | 2nd–5th MCP, full ext |
| Lumbar spine | lat flex and ER | ext (facet joints) |
| Hip | flex, abd, IR | combined ext, IR, and abd |
| Knee | flex, ext | full ext |
| Ankle (talocrural joint) | PF, DF | full DF |
| IP | flex, ext | full ext |

Data from Magee DJ: *Orthopedic Physical Assessment*, 3rd ed. Philadelphia, WB Saunders, 1997, and Maitland GD: *Peripheral Manipulation*, 3rd ed. Boston, Butterworth-Heinemann, 1991.

# APPENDIX G

## Radiology

I. Suggested methodology for evaluating radiographs: observe radiographs methodically, looking for abnormalities in the following order (ABCs):

A: alignment (of bones/vertebrae; no displacement/ deformity?)

B: bony changes (changes in density, Fxs, spurring, sclerosis)

C: cartilage/disc space (joint space, lack thereof, indicating DJD or DDD)

S: soft tissue (some soft tissues such as the psoas major can be seen on radiographs, and abnormalities such as an abscess or hemorrhaging may be identified)

II. Radiologic techniques for specific conditions: some techniques are better suited for identifying specific conditions than others

Radiography: Fx, OCD/osteochondral defects, femoral head dislocation/dysplasia, joint dislocation

CT scan: HNP, vertebral body abnormalities, abscess or neoplasm, intraarticular Fx fragments, pelvis fracture, meniscal tears

MRI: soft tissue lesions (lig, tendon, and muscle tears/ ruptures, soft tissue tumors), meniscus tears, spinal cord anomalies, avascular necrosis of the femoral head, HNP

Bone scan: stress Fxs, skeletal metastasis/bone tumors, osteomyelitis

Myelography: visualization of the spinal cord, nerve roots, and thecal sac

III. Before ordering a radiologic examination, ask yourself the following questions as put forth by Dr. John R. Thornbury:

1. Is this examination going to affect my diagnostic certainty about the differential diagnosis I am considering, and if so, how much?

2. Will the information expected to be provided by the examination change my diagnostic thinking enough so that it will significantly affect my choice of treatment?

## Bibliography

James H. Swain: ABCS of radiology. Presented in a class entitled Radiology for Physical Therapists and adapted from Scheurger SR: Introduction to critical review of roentgenograms. Phys Ther 68:1114–1120, 1988.

Thornbury JR: Clinical decision making in use of imaging examinations. In Kuhns LR, Thornbury JR, Fryback DG (eds): *Decisions in Imaging*. Chicago, Year Book Medical Publishers, 1989.

Parker MD: *Introduction to Radiology*. Philadelphia, JB Lippincott, 1985.

# APPENDIX H

Physical Agent and Modalities

| Physical Agent | Indications | Contraindications | Notes |
|---|---|---|---|
| Superficial heat (depth of penetration of various techniques for superficial heat is approx 1 cm) | Pain modulation<br>Reduce joint stiffness<br>Alleviate muscle guarding/ "spasm"<br>Increase ROM<br>Increase blood flow | Over areas of impaired temperature sensation, impaired circulation, active hemorrhage, or acute inflammation<br>Tumor<br>Pt who cannot verbally tell you that it is too hot<br>Skin infection | Methods of superficial heat include<br>*Hot packs (hydrocollator)*: do not have Pt lie on hot pack; wrap pack in 6–8 towel thickness<br>*Paraffin*: commonly used for hands and feet, also used to moisturize and increase pliability of scar from burn or injury<br>*Fluidotherapy*: also used to desensitize skin after peripheral nerve injuries or any type of hyperesthesia<br>*Radiation (infrared lamp)*: intensity affected by inverse square and cosine law<br>*Hydrotherapy*: additional uses include debridement, over painful scars, adhesions, arthritis, as warm-up for exercises, relaxation |

| Superficial cold | | |
|---|---|---|
| Acute musculoskeletal trauma | Over areas of impaired temperature sensation or impaired circulation | Methods of superficial cold include Cold pack/crushed ice pack |
| Reduce spasticity | Cold hypersensitivity | Ice massage |
| Pain modulation | Certain cardiovascular diseases | Ice immersion |
| Increase ROM | Superficial nerve trunk, especially applying pressure/compression | Cold compression |
| Myofascial pain syndrome | Certain rheumatoid conditions | Vapocoolant sprays |
| | | Types of cold hypersensitivity include cold urticaria, cryoglobinemia, cold intolerance, vasospastic disease, cold hemoglobinuria |
| | | Types of cardiovascular disease that could be adversely affected by cold: Raynaud's phenomenon, HTN, coronary artery disease |

*Continued* ▶

| Physical Agent | Indications | Contraindications | Notes |
|---|---|---|---|
| Short wave diathermy (heating modality) | Pain modulation | In presence of pacemakers or other implanted stimulators | Methods of short wave diathermy |
| | Reduce joint stiffness | Over areas of decreased sensation | *Capacitive:* depth of penetration approx 1 cm. Tissues with high electrical resistance are selectively heated (e.g., fat, skin, ligament, capsule, cartilage). |
| | Alleviate muscle guarding/spasm | Over eyes (heating of eye fluid) | |
| | Increase ROM | Metal objects in area to be treated (e.g., jewelry, metal implants) | Caution: nylon or foam rubber in field may burn. |
| | Increase blood flow | Over pelvic area of female Pt during menstruation | *Inductive:* depth of penetration approx 3 cm. Tissues with high magnetic resistance are selectively heated (e.g., muscle, blood, sweat). |
| | | Over moist wound dressings | |
| | | Over tumors | Caution: moisture (sweat or exudate from wound) in field absorbs energy and may burn Pt |
| | | Over testes of male Pt | |
| | | Over active hemorrhage or acute inflammation | |
| | | Over ischemic tissue | |
| | | Over open growth plate/epiphysis in children | |
| | | During pregnancy | |

| | | | |
|---|---|---|---|
| Pulsed electromagnetic field | Soft tissue injury<br>Cutaneous wound healing | In presence of pacemakers and implanted stimulators<br>Over tumors<br>During pregnancy<br>If mean power approaches 80 watts, include contraindications for thermal effects as above for short wave diathermy | |
| Laser | Wound healing<br>Pain modulation<br>Scar tissue reduction<br>Edema and inflammation | Into, over, or around eyes<br>During pregnancy<br>In pt who is photosensitive | HeNe penetrates 2–5 mm<br>GaAs penetrates 1–2 cm<br>HeNe, indirect effects to 8–10 mm<br>GaAs, indirect effects to 5 cm |

*Continued* ▶

| Physical Agent | Indications | Contraindications | Notes |
|---|---|---|---|
| Ultraviolet light | Acne | Over or into the unprotected eye | Used mainly for dermatology patients |
| | Aseptic and septic wounds | When pt is taking drugs or eating foods that cause hypersensitivity to UV radiation (e.g., gold therapy, sulfa drugs, insulin, thyroxine, quinine, tetracycline, eggs [sulfa], lobster [sulfa], aniline dyes [in coal tar for psoriasis]) | Depth of penetration is epidermis |
| | Folliculitis | | |
| | Pityriasis rosea | | |
| | Tinea capitum | | |
| | Sinusitis | | |
| | | Porphyria | |
| | | Pellagra | |
| | | Sarcoidosis | |
| | | Lupus erythematosus | |
| | | Xeroderma pigmentosum | |
| | | Active and progressive pulmonary tuberculosis | |
| | | Acute psoriasis | |
| | | Advanced arteriosclerosis | |
| | | General dermatitis | |
| | | Hyperthyroidism | |

| Ultrasound | Do not apply over | Types of ultrasound |
|---|---|---|
| *Thermal effects:* joint contracture, scar tissue mobilization, chronic bursitis, chronic tendinitis, muscle guarding/spasm–pain cycle<br><br>*Nonthermal effects:* wound/tissue healing, plantar warts, Fx healing, detecting stress Fxs | Areas of impaired pain/temperature sensation<br>Areas of reduced circulation<br>Thrombophlebitis<br>Eyes<br>Testes/ovaries<br>Heart<br>Pacemaker<br>Malignant tissue<br>Spinal cord<br>Cervical/stellate ganglia<br>Epiphyseal areas of children, abdominal region of females during the reproductive years or immediately after menses<br><br>Do not apply during pregnancy | 1.0 MHz: penetrates approx 4–6 cm<br>3.0 MHz: penetrates approx 1–2 cm<br><br>Pulsed ultrasound eliminates thermal effect by using 20–50% duty cycle. Heating depends on the temporal average:<br><br>$$\text{duty cycle} = \frac{\text{on time}}{\text{on time + off time}} \times 100$$<br><br>Ultrasound has affinity for tissues containing high protein content<br><br>It is recommended that ultrasound be limited to 14 treatments |

*Continued* ▶

| Physical Agent | Indications | Contraindications | Notes |
|---|---|---|---|
| **Electrotherapy** | | | |
| Pulsatile (mono-, bi-, and polyphasic) | Analgesia | Demand-type cardiac pacemaker | If Pt is able to participate, active therapeutic exercise is often better at accomplishing goals of many indications listed here |
| | Muscle re-education | Cardiac arrhythmia | |
| | Prevent atrophy | Over carotid artery | |
| | Spasticity reduction | Hypersensitive patients | |
| | Cutaneous wound healing | Pregnancy | |
| | Fx healing | Patient with central venous line | |
| | Scoliosis | Adjacent to or distal to area of thrombophlebitis | |
| | Orthotic substitution | Over area of abnormal skin | |
| | Reduce swelling | | |
| | Increase blood flow | | |
| | Ventilation (phrenic driving) | | |
| Direct current | Iontophoresis | Same as above | Caution: direct current can burn skin |
| | Wound healing | | Aids debridement |

## Bibliography

Griffin JE, Karselis TC: *Physical Agents for Physical Therapists*, 2nd ed. Springfield, IL, Charles C Thomas, 1988.

Lehmann JF (ed): *Therapeutic Heat and Cold*, 4th ed. Baltimore, Williams & Wilkins, 1990.

Nelson RM, Currier DP: *Clinical Electrotherapy*, 2nd ed. Norwalk, CT, Appleton & Lange, 1991.

Prentice WE: *Therapeutic Modalities in Sports Medicine*, 3rd ed. St. Louis, Mosby–Year Book, 1994.

# APPENDIX I
Types of Traction

| Type of Traction | Indications | Contraindications | Notes |
|---|---|---|---|
| Cervical or lumbar traction | Disc protrusion<br>Degenerative disc/joint<br>Disease (especially that resulting in foraminal encroachment)<br>Joint hypomobility<br>Facet impingement<br>Muscle spasm/guarding | *Absolute contraindications:*<br>Spinal tumor<br>Spinal infection<br>Vertebral artery disease (cervical traction only)<br>Trauma where Fx has not been excluded<br>*Relative contraindications:*<br>Acute strains/sprains<br>Acute inflammatory conditions (e.g., rheumatoid arthritis)<br>Joint instability (e.g., during pregnancy, prolonged steroid use, Down's syndrome)<br>Osteoporosis<br>Hiatal hernia | Use precaution in presence of any contraindication (absolute or relative). Sources differ on what is considered an absolute or relative contraindication. Remember, above all else, **DO NO HARM!** |

## Bibliography

Kisner C, Colby LA: *Therapeutic Exercise: Foundations and Techniques*, 2nd ed. Philadelphia, FA Davis, 1990.

Saunders HD, Saunders R: *Evaluation, Treatment, and Prevention of Musculoskeletal Disorders: Spine*, 3rd ed, Vol 1. Chaska, MN Educational Opportunities, 1995.

# APPENDIX J

Normal Values for Commonly Encountered
Laboratory Results

| Component | Normal Range |
|---|---|
| **Blood** | |
| Albumin | 3.1–4.3 g/dL |
| Bicarbonate ($HCO_3^-$) | 22–26 mEq/L (nonpregnant adult) |
| Cholesterol (total) | <200 mg/dL |
|   HDL cholesterol | 44–45 mg/dL male |
| | 55 mg/dL female |
|   LDL cholesterol | <130 mg/dL (desirable) |
| Cortisol | |
|   8 AM (client at rest) | 5–25 μg/dL |
|   8 PM | <10 μg/dL |
| CPK (CK II) | <10 U/L |
| Creatinine | 0.6–1.5 mg/dL male |
| | 0.6–1.1 mg/dL female |
| Creatine kinase | 60–100 U/L (male) |
|   Total | 40–150 U/L (female) |
| Erythrocyte count | 4.6–5.9 million/mm³ (male) |
| | 4.2–5.4 million/mm³ (female) |
| Glucose (fasting) | 70–110 mg/dL |
| Hematocrit (Hct) | 0.45–0.52% (male) |
| | 0.37–0.48% (female) |
| Hemoglobin (Hgb) | 13–18 g/dL (male) |
| | 12–16 g/dL (female) |
| Iron | 80–180 μg/dL (male) |
| | 60–160 μg/dL (female) |
| Leukocyte count | 4300–10,800/mm³ |
| pH of blood | 7.35–7.45 (arterial) |
| | 7.30–7.41 (venous) |
| $P_{O_2}$ (blood gas) | 75–100 mm Hg |

*Continued* ▶

J | NORMAL VALUES FOR COMMONLY ENCOUNTERED LABORATORY RESULTS

| Component | Normal Range |
|---|---|
| **Blood** *Continued* | |
| $P_{CO_2}$ (blood gas) | 35–45 mm Hg (arterial) |
| | 41–51 mm Hg (venous) |
| | (slightly lower in females) |
| Platelet count | 150,000–350,000/mm$^3$ |
| Thyroxine, total (T$_4$) | 4.0–11.0 μg/dL |
| Triiodothyronine, total (T$_3$) | 75–220 ng/dL |
| Thyroid-stimulating hormone (TSH) | 0.5–5.0 μU/mL |
| Triglycerides | 40–150 mg/dL (nonpregnant adult; |
| | females slightly lower) |
| | 130–135 mg/dL (>65 y) |
| **Coagulation Tests** | |
| Prothrombin time (PT) | Control 8.8–11.6 sec (± 2 sec) |
| Partial thromboplastin time (PTT) | 24–37 sec for activated PTT |
| | 60–90 sec if not activated |
| **Erythrocyte Sedimentation Rate** | |
| Westergren method | |
| Adult | |
| Male | 1–13 mm/h |
| Female | 1–20 mm/h |
| Pregnancy | 44–114 mm/h |
| Senior adult (< 50 y) | |
| Male | 1–20 mm/h |
| Female | 1–30 mm/h |
| Child | 1–13 mm/h |
| Wintrobe method | |
| Adult | |
| Male | 1–9 mm/h |
| Female | 1–20 mm/h |

Corbett JB: *Laboratory Tests and Diagnostic Procedures with Nursing Diagnoses*, 4th ed. Stamford, CT, Appleton & Lange, 1996.

# APPENDIX K

## Abbreviations and Definitions

This list contains abbreviations and definitions specific to this text. Most facilities or practices have their own lists of approved abbreviations, and the facility's list should take precedence in the event of a conflict.

AAA: abdominal aortic aneurysm
AAROM: active assisted range of motion
abd: abduction
AC: acromioclavicular
ACL: anterior cruciate ligament
add: adduction
ADLs: activities of daily living
AGG: aggravating factors or activities that increase Sx
AKA: above-knee amputation
AP: anteroposterior (e.g., anteroposterior glides)
APL: abductor pollicis longus
approx: approximately
AROM: active range of motion
ASIS: anterior superior iliac spine
ATFL: anterior talofibular ligament
ATNR: asymmetric tonic neck reflex
ATTL: anterior tibiotalar ligament
athetosis: slow, writhing, involuntary movements of limbs and facial muscles
B/B: bowel/bladder (e.g., frequency, urgency, retention)
BKA: below-knee amputation
BW: birth weight
CFL: calcaneofibular ligament
chorea: abrupt, involuntary movements of limb and face muscles
clonus: alternate involuntary muscular contraction and relaxation of rapid succession in response to quick stretch
C/O: complains of
coxa vara: decreased angle between femoral neck and shaft (<120 deg)
coxa valga: increased angle between femoral neck and shaft (>135 deg)
crepitus: a grinding/cracking/popping sound or sensation in joints associated with active range of motion
CT: computed tomography
DDD: degenerative disc disease
deg: degrees

dermatome: area of the skin innervated by a single dorsal nerve root

DF: dorsiflexion

DIP: distal interphalangeal joint

DJD: degenerative joint disease

DP: dorsal pedal pulse

duration: duration of symptoms

Dx: diagnosis

EASE: easing factors, activities, or positions that decrease symptoms

EBL: estimated blood loss

ECG: electrocardiograph

EPB: extensor pollicis brevis muscle

ER: external rotation

ev: eversion

exostosis: excess bone deposition

ext: extension

FCU: flexor carpi ulnaris

FDP: flexor digitorum profundus

$FEV_1$: forced expiratory volume at 1 second (volume of gas that can be forcefully expelled from the lungs in 1 second—normally about 80%)

flex: flexion

FOOSH: fall on outstretched hand

FPL: flexor pollicis longus

FRC: functional residual capacity (volume of air in the lungs at the resting end-expiratory level)

FWB: full weight bearing

Fx: fracture

genu recurvatum: excessively hyperextended knee

GMMT: gross manual muscle testing

HNP: herniated nucleus pulposus

H/O: history of

HTN: hypertension

Hx: history

inv: inversion

IP: interphalangeal joint

IR: internal rotation

ITB: iliotibial band

lat: lateral

LBP: low back pain

LCL: lateral collateral ligament

LE: lower extremity

LT: light touch

MCL: medial collateral ligament

MCP: metacarpal phalangeal joint

MD: medical doctor

med: medial

Meds: medications patient is taking

MHx: medical history

MMT: manual muscle testing/strength testing

MOI: mechanism of injury if symptoms result from trauma

MP: metacarpal phalangeal joint

MRI: magnetic resonance imaging

MSR: muscle stretch reflex

nature of pain: constant or intermittent, ache/sharp/burning/ stabbing, difference in time of day (morning or evening); 24-hour behavior

NSAIDs: nonsteroidal antiinflammatory drugs

NWB: non–weight-bearing

nystagmus: involuntary rapid eye movement

OA: osteoarthritis

OCD: osteochondritis dissecans

onset: onset of symptoms (insidious or trauma)

ORIF: open reduction internal fixation

PA: posteroanterior (e.g., posteroanterior glide mobilization)

PACVP: posteroanterior central vertebral pressure

PAIVM: passive accessory intervertebral motion

PAUVP: posteroanterior unilateral vertebral pressure

PCL: posterior cruciate ligament

Pes cavus: excessively high arched foot

Pes planus: excessively low arched foot

PF: plantar flexion

PFT: pulmonary function test

PIP: proximal interphalangeal

plica: remnants of the embryonic synovial membrane that usually regress in the adult

PMHx: past medical history

PPIVM: passive physiologic intervertebral movement

PQ: pronator quadratus

PRE: progressive resistive exercise

PROM: passive range of motion

PSHx: past surgical history

PSIS: posterior superior iliac spine

Pt: patient

PT: posterior tibial artery pulse

PTFL: posterior talofibular ligament

PTS: prone to sit

PTTL: posterior tibiotalar ligament

PWB: partial weight bearing

rales: abnormal breath sounds, a bubbling noise heard in the chest while breathing in

RCL: radial collateral ligament

REIL: repeated extension in lying

REIS: repeated extension in standing

RF: rheumatoid factor

RFIL: repeated flexion in lying

RFIS: repeated flexion in standing

R/O: rule out

ROM: range of motion

rot: rotation

Rx: treatment

SAID: specific adaptation to imposed demand

SC: sternoclavicular

sclerotome: the area of a bone innervated from a single spinal segment

SCM: sternocleidomastoid muscle

SI: sacroiliac

SLR: straight-leg raise

spondylosis: vertebral ankylosis; any degenerative changes in the spine

spondylolisthesis: forward displacement of a vertebra over a lower segment, usually of the fourth or fifth lumbar vertebra, caused by a developmental defect in the pars interarticularis

spondylolysis: fracture of the posterior arch of the vertebra at the pars interarticularis but no translation of the vertebral body

SQ: special questions, such as about unrelenting night pain, bowel or bladder symptoms, saddle anesthesia, unexplained weight loss, or history of diabetes/cancer/osteoarthritis/rheumatoid arthritis/osteoporosis/hypertension/cardiac disorders

STNR: symmetric tonic neck reflex

Sx: symptom(s)

TCL: tibiocalcaneal ligament

TFL: tensor fascia latae

TFM: transverse friction massage

THL: transverse humeral ligament

TNL: tibionavicular ligament

TOCS: thoracic outlet compression syndrome

TTP: tender to palpation

UCL: ulnar collateral ligament

UE: upper extremity

UTI: urinary tract infection

VA: vertebral artery (tests for VA insufficiency)

VC: vital capacity (maximal volume of air measured on complete expiration after full inspiration)

VMO: vastus medialis obliquus

$V_t$: tidal volume (volume of air that is inspired or expired in a single breath during regular breathing)

# INDEX

Note: Page numbers followed by the letter t refer to tables.

INDEX

INDEX